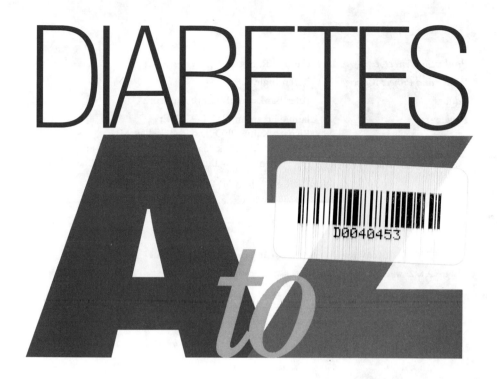

DIABETES
A to Z

What You Need to Know
About Diabetes – Simply Put

Third Edition

△. American Diabetes Association

Production Director	Carolyn R. Segree
Writer and Project Manager	Karen Ingle
Editors	Peter Banks and Sherrye Landrum
Reviewers	Janine Freeman, RD, LD, CDE; Richard Kahn, PhD; David B. Kelley, MD; Barbara J. Maschak-Carey, RNCS, MSN, CDE; and Virginia Peragallo-Dittko, RN, MA, CDE
Designer/Desktop Publishing	Harlowe Typography, Inc.
Cover Design	Wickham & Associates
Illustrations	Duckwall Productions

Library of Congress Cataloging-in-Publication Data

Diabetes A to Z: what you need to know about diabetes : simply put. — 3rd ed.
      p.   cm.
    Includes index.
    ISBN 0-945448-96-1   (pbk.)
    1. Diabetes—Popular works. I. American Diabetes Association.
RC660.4.D526 1997
616.4'62—dc21   97-30806
                                                CIP

Printed in the United States of America

The suggestions and information contained in this publication are generally consistent with the Clinical Practice Recommendations and other policies of the American Diabetes Association, but they do not represent the policy or position of the Association or any of its boards or committees. Reasonable steps have been taken to ensure the accuracy of the information presented. However, the American Diabetes Association cannot ensure the safety or efficacy of any product or service described in this publication. Individuals are advised to consult a physician or other appropriate health-care professional before undertaking any diet or exercise program or taking any medication referred to in this publication. Professionals must use and apply their own professional judgment, experience, and training and should not rely solely on the information contained in this publication before prescribing any diet, exercise, or medication. The American Diabetes Association—its officers, directors, employees, volunteers, and members—assumes no responsibility or liability for personal or other injury, loss, or damage that may result from the suggestions or information in this publication.

American Diabetes Association
1660 Duke Street, Alexandria, VA 22314

Table of Contents

Foreword

Maybe you've just been diagnosed with diabetes or maybe you've had diabetes for years. Perhaps a member of your family or a friend has diabetes. Whatever your situation, you want to find out all you can about the disease. That's where *Diabetes A to Z* can help. It explains everything you need to know about diabetes in clear, simple terms.

Diabetes A to Z is an encyclopedia of diabetes. It is arranged alphabetically, so you can more easily find the information you need. You may also enjoy just browsing from entry to entry.

The information in each entry will help you understand how to balance your diabetes care with a full and active lifestyle. You will even find helpful tips on coping with the social and emotional challenges of day-to-day life with diabetes.

We hope *Diabetes A to Z* helps you understand your diabetes better, so that you can live a longer, happier, and healthier life.

Frank Vinicor, MD, MPH
Past President, American Diabetes Association

Alcohol

Drinking small amounts of alcohol may be okay if you have good control of your diabetes, don't have complications, and fit the alcohol into your meal plan. But drinking alcohol on an empty stomach can cause low blood glucose if you then exercise or if you are taking diabetes pills or insulin.

ALCOHOL AND LOW BLOOD GLUCOSE

Insulin lowers your blood glucose. Diabetes pills (except metformin, acarbose, and troglitazone) make your body release more insulin to lower blood glucose. Exercise makes your insulin work better at lowering blood glucose.

Usually, if your blood glucose drops too low, the liver puts more glucose into the blood. (The liver has its own supply of glucose, called glycogen.) But when alcohol, a toxin, is in the body, the liver wants to get rid of it first. While the liver is taking care of the alcohol, it may let blood glucose drop to dangerous levels.

To avoid low blood glucose

- Eat something when you drink alcohol.
- Check your blood glucose before, during, and after drinking. Alcohol can lower blood glucose as long as 8 to 12 hours after your last drink.

- Plan ahead how much you will drink. Don't drink more than is included in your meal plan.

If you have low blood glucose after you drink, people might smell the alcohol and think you are drunk. The signs are the same. Tell them you have low blood glucose. Tell them what they need to do to help you take care of it. Wear a medical I.D. bracelet stating that you have diabetes. This will help in case you can't talk.

If you drink and then drive when you have low blood glucose, you may be pulled over for drunk driving. You may even have an accident. When you drink—even a small amount—let someone else drive. Pick a responsible person ahead of time.

ALCOHOL AND COMPLICATIONS

Alcohol can worsen nerve damage, eye diseases, high blood pressure, and high blood fats. If you have any of these problems, ask your doctor how much alcohol, if any, is safe for you to drink.

ALCOHOL AND YOUR MEAL PLAN

Work with a dietitian to include your favorite drink in your meal plan. Be aware that regular beer, sweet wines, and wine coolers will raise your blood glucose more than light beer, dry wines, and liquors (such as vodka, scotch, and whiskey) because they contain more carbohydrate.

Carbohydrate is the main nutrient that raises blood glucose. If you are watching your weight, be aware that alcoholic drinks can have anywhere from 60 to 300 calories each.

To cut calories

- Use 80 proof in place of 100 proof alcohol. The lower the proof number, the less alcohol. Each gram of alcohol has 7 calories.
- Put less liquor in your drink.
- Use no-calorie mixers, such as club soda or water.
- Choose light beer over regular beer.

- Choose dry wine over sweet or fruity wines and wine coolers.
- Try a wine spritzer made with a small amount of wine and club soda.

Drink	Serving	Calories	Exchanges
Liquor	1.5 oz	107	2.5 Fats
Dry table wine	3.0 oz	68	1.5 Fats
Wine cooler	12 oz	196	3 Fats, 1 Starch
Regular beer	12 oz	151	2 Fats, 1 Starch
Light beer	12 oz	97	2 Fats

Blood Fats

Fats are part of every cell in your body. Fats include cholesterol and triglycerides. Both cholesterol and triglycerides are made by your body. You can also get them from the animal foods you eat.

Your body uses cholesterol to build cell walls and to make certain vitamins and hormones. Your body uses triglycerides as stored fat. Stored fat keeps you warm, protects your body's organs, and gives you energy reserves.

Cholesterol and triglycerides travel through your body in your blood. These two blood fats can only travel by being carried. They are carried by lipoproteins (*lipo* means fat). Three kinds of lipoproteins are

1. Very-low-density lipoprotein (VLDL). VLDL carries triglycerides, cholesterol, and other fats. VLDL drops off triglycerides and other fats in fat tissue. VLDL then becomes LDL.

2. Low-density lipoprotein (LDL). LDL carries cholesterol to parts of the body that need it. Along the way, LDL cholesterol can stick to blood vessel walls. Cholesterol on blood vessel walls can lead to blood vessel disease. The less LDL in your blood, the better.

3. High-density lipoprotein (HDL). HDL carries cholesterol away from the blood vessel walls to the liver. The liver breaks the cholesterol down and sends it out of the body. The more HDL in your blood, the better.

People with diabetes often have high blood fat levels. High blood fat levels put you at risk for heart disease, heart attack, and stroke. If you want to reduce your risk, first find out what your blood fat levels are.

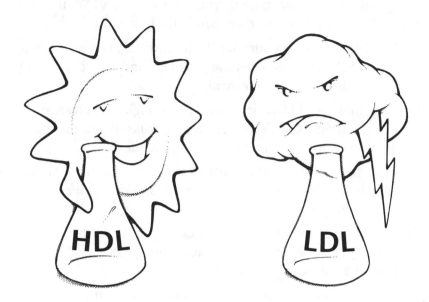

THE HEALTHIEST BLOOD FAT LEVELS ARE

- Total cholesterol under 200 mg/dl
- LDL cholesterol under 130 mg/dl
- HDL cholesterol over 35 mg/dl
- Triglycerides under 200 mg/dl

If your blood fat levels match these, great! If your blood fat levels do not match these, try the following steps.

TO IMPROVE BLOOD FAT LEVELS

- First, control your diabetes. Controlling your diabetes means keeping your blood glucose in a range set by your doctor. When your diabetes is out of control, none of the other steps will help.

- If you are overweight, lose a few pounds. Extra weight makes it harder to control blood glucose and raises total cholesterol. Besides, losing weight raises your good HDL cholesterol.

- Start cutting back on all fat (see Diet). Your liver uses the fat you eat to make VLDL. The more fat you eat, the more VLDL the liver makes. More VLDL means more bad LDL cholesterol.

- Replace saturated fats (butter, lard) with unsaturated fats (most vegetable oils). Saturated fats raise your LDL and total cholesterol levels. Unsaturated fats lower them.

- Eat high-cholesterol foods less often. Foods high in cholesterol include organ meats, such as liver, and egg yolks. If you eat eggs every day, try cutting back to three or four a week.

- Eat foods high in fiber. Some types of fiber help remove cholesterol from the body. Oats, beans, peas, fresh fruits, and brown rice are great fiber choices.

- Take a hike or go for a walk. Aerobic exercises, such as brisk walking, jogging, swimming, and skiing, raise your good HDL cholesterol. Find exercises you enjoy.

- If you smoke, cut down or quit. Smoking lowers your good HDL cholesterol.

Have your blood fat levels tested at least once a year, or more often if your doctor recommends it.

Blood Glucose

The foods you eat are broken down into glucose by your body. Glucose is a sugar. Glucose travels through your blood to your cells. Cells use glucose for energy. To get inside your cells, glucose needs the help of insulin.

In people with diabetes, there is a problem with the insulin. Sometimes there is no insulin (see Type 1 Diabetes). Other times there is insulin, but the body has trouble using it or there isn't enough of it (see Type 2 Diabetes).

When insulin is not able to do its job, glucose cannot get into the cells. Instead, glucose collects in the blood. The amount of glucose in your blood is called your blood glucose level.

Too much glucose in the blood is called hyperglycemia or high blood glucose. Too little glucose in the blood is called hypoglycemia or low blood glucose. Blood glucose that has gone up too far or down too low can make you feel ill and harm your body (see Blood Glucose, High; Blood Glucose, Low).

To feel good and stay healthy, keep your blood glucose between the highs and lows—in a range your doctor advises. See the table on the next page.

Keeping blood glucose in your ideal range and avoiding the highs and lows takes some effort. You can do it by balancing food, activity, and diabetes pills or insulin. One of your best tools is blood glucose tests. Here are some tips for success.

IDEAL BLOOD GLUCOSE RANGES FOR PEOPLE WITH DIABETES

Time	Glucose (mg/dl)
In the morning, before breakfast	80 to 120
Before meals	80 to 120
1 to 2 hours after a meal	Less than 180
At bedtime	100 to 140
At 3:00 A.M.	Over 80

These ranges are based on blood tests you do at home (see Blood Glucose, Self-Tests) rather than lab tests. These may not be the best ranges for you. Talk to your doctor about what your ranges should be.

FOOD

- Follow your meal plan (see Meal Planning).
- Include snacks in your meal plan only if your doctor or dietitian recommends it.
- Eat meals and snacks around the same times each day.
- Don't skip or delay meals or snacks.
- Eat the same amounts of foods from day to day.
- If you take insulin, ask your doctor or nurse how to adjust your dose when you want to eat more or less than usual.

ACTIVITY

- Follow your exercise program.
- If you take insulin or diabetes pills and you are going to exercise for more than 1 hour, eat snacks. Examples of snacks are a piece of fruit, 1/2 cup of juice, 1/2 bagel, or a small roll. Talk with a dietitian or diabetes educator about how much and when to eat.
- Be sure to check your blood glucose levels after exercise. Exercise lowers blood glucose for as long as 10 to 24 hours afterward.

- If you take insulin, ask your doctor or nurse if you need to adjust your dose for exercise.

DIABETES PILLS OR INSULIN

- Take insulin or diabetes pills as your doctor or nurse has directed.
- Talk with your doctor about changing your insulin or diabetes pills if your blood glucose levels are not in your ideal range. Perhaps a different dosage or type of insulin or pills would work better for you.
- If you take insulin, ask your nurse or diabetes educator about the best places to inject it. Some people find that taking their insulin in the same place keeps blood glucose steadier.
- Consider an insulin pump. Pumps imitate the natural release of insulin better than shots do (see Insulin Pumps).

TESTING

- Test your blood glucose often. If you test once a day, consider two or three times a day.
- Test your blood glucose if

  You ate too much or too little food.

  You delayed or skipped a meal or snack.

  You are sick.

  You are under stress.

  You did not take your insulin or diabetes pills.

  You took too much insulin

  You took too many diabetes pills.

  You did not do your usual exercise.

  You exercised harder or longer than usual.

Blood Glucose, High

Too much glucose in the blood is called hyperglycemia or high blood glucose. High blood glucose is one of the signs of diabetes. Over time, high blood glucose can damage your eyes, kidneys, heart, nerves, and blood vessels.

CAUSES OF HIGH BLOOD GLUCOSE

- You ate too much food.
- You took too little insulin.
- You did not take your insulin.
- You took too few diabetes pills.
- You did not take your diabetes pills.
- You are sick.
- You feel stressed.
- You skipped your usual exercise.

High blood glucose is harder to sense than low blood glucose. If your glucose is very high, you may feel some of the following signs.

SIGNS OF HIGH BLOOD GLUCOSE

- Headache
- Blurry vision
- Thirst

- Hunger
- Upset stomach
- Frequent urination
- Dry, itchy skin
- Fruity smell on breath

You may not be able to tell that your glucose is too high by these signs alone. The only sure way to know is *to test your blood glucose* (see Blood Glucose, Self-Tests). Your glucose reading will help you decide what to do.

TO TREAT HIGH BLOOD GLUCOSE

If your blood glucose is between 180 and 240

1. Do as your doctor has advised you. You may have been told to try one of the following:
   - A small extra dose of Regular (short-acting) insulin
   - A walk or some other exercise
   - A smaller upcoming snack

2. Check your blood glucose again after 1 to 2 hours.

If your blood glucose is over 240 mg/dl

Test your urine for ketones. High blood glucose can lead to a buildup of ketones. Ketones are made when your body burns fat instead of glucose for energy. If not treated, ketones can harm your body. Call your doctor if there are ketones in your urine.

If your blood glucose is over 350 mg/dl

Test your urine for ketones. Call your doctor right away.

If your blood glucose is over 500 mg/dl

Test your urine for ketones. Call your doctor right away. Your doctor will probably send you to a hospital. If you can't reach your doctor, go to a hospital.

Blood Glucose, Low

Too little glucose in the blood is called hypoglycemia or low blood glucose. Low blood glucose may occur if you use insulin or take diabetes pills (other than metformin, acarbose, or troglitazone). If not treated, low blood glucose can make you pass out. At worst, low blood glucose may cause seizures, coma, and even death.

CAUSES OF LOW BLOOD GLUCOSE

- You ate too little food.
- You ate too few carbohydrates.
- You delayed a meal or snack.
- You skipped a meal or snack.
- You exercised harder or longer than usual.
- You took too much insulin or too many diabetes pills.
- You are sick.
- You drank alcohol on an empty stomach.

WARNING SIGNS OF LOW BLOOD GLUCOSE

There are many warning signs of low blood glucose. Your own signs may be different from what someone else feels. Learn your early warning signs of low blood glucose. Share your signs with someone who can help you notice them.

WARNING SIGNS

Your signs may not be on this list.

Angry	Irritable	Sick to stomach
Anxious	Light-headed	Sleepy
Clammy	Nervous	Stubborn
Clumsy	Numb	Sweaty
Confused	Pale	Tense
Hungry	Sad	Tired
Impatient	Shaky	Weak

You may also have blurry vision, a dry mouth, a headache, or a pounding heart. When any of your warning signs occur, you need to treat low blood glucose right away.

TO TREAT YOURSELF FOR LOW BLOOD GLUCOSE

1. Test your blood glucose with a meter if you can (see Blood Glucose, Self-Tests).

If it is under 70 mg/dl

   Go to steps 2 and 3. If you can't test, go to steps 2 and 4.

2. Eat or drink something with about 15 grams (1/2 oz) of carbohydrate. Foods with 15 grams of carbohydrate are listed in the table on p. 14.

3. Wait 15 to 20 minutes, then test again.

If your blood glucose is still below 70 mg/dl

   Repeat steps 2 and 3. If you have repeated steps 2 and 3 and your blood glucose is still below 70 mg/dl, call your doctor or have someone take you to a hospital emergency room. You may need help to treat it. Or something else may be causing the signs.

If your blood glucose is over 70 mg/dl

Stop drinking and/or eating foods listed in the table. You may still feel the signs of low blood glucose even after your blood glucose is back up. Go to step 4.

4. If your next meal is more than an hour away, eat a small snack of carbohydrate and protein. Try a slice of bread with reduced-fat peanut butter or six crackers with low-fat cheese.

TREAT LOW BLOOD GLUCOSE WITH ONE OF THESE FOODS

1/2 cup (4 oz) of fruit juice

1/3 can (4 oz) of a regular (not sugar-free) soft drink

1 cup (8 oz) of skim milk

2 tablespoons of raisins (40 to 50)

3 graham crackers

4 teaspoons of granulated sugar

6 saltine crackers

6 1/2-inch sugar cubes

1 tablespoon of honey or syrup

Glucose tablets or gel (dose is printed on the package)

HAVING SOMEONE ELSE TREAT YOUR LOW GLUCOSE

Sometimes you will not be able to treat low blood glucose yourself. Maybe you do not notice your signs. Or maybe low blood glucose has made you too confused to treat yourself. Whatever the reason, teach someone else *ahead of time* to do it.

Keep foods to treat low blood glucose near you at all times. Place a small box of juice in your desk drawer at work or at school. Put glucose tablets or gel in your purse or coat pocket and in the glove compartment of your car. Tell others where you keep them.

If you take insulin, get a glucagon emergency kit. Your doctor can prescribe one. Glucagon is a hormone that is made in the pancreas. Glucagon makes the liver release glucose into the blood.

A glucagon kit comes with a syringe of glucagon and instructions on how to use it. Keep the kit with you. Tell family, friends, and co-workers where you keep it. You or your doctor or a nurse can teach them how to use it.

If you can swallow

Have someone get you to eat or drink something with carbohydrate in it.

If you cannot swallow or if you pass out

Have someone

1. Inject you with glucagon in the front of the thigh or the shoulder muscle.

2. Turn you on your side. This will keep you from choking if you throw up from the glucagon. (Some people feel sick to their stomach after glucagon.)

Once you are alert

3. Eat a snack of carbohydrate that's easy on your stomach. Try six saltine crackers. Follow it up with a snack of protein, such as a slice of turkey breast or low-fat cheese.

4. Test your blood glucose every 30 to 60 minutes to make sure low blood glucose is not coming back.

If you cannot swallow and glucagon is not available OR
if you cannot swallow and nobody knows how to use glucagon

Have someone

1. Call 911 for an ambulance.

2. Moisten his or her fingertip. Dip the fingertip in table sugar. Rub his or her sugar-coated finger tip against the inside of your cheek until the sugar dissolves, being careful to keep the finger away from your teeth. (If you go into a seizure, you may bite the finger.)

OR

Have someone open a tube of cake frosting and insert the open end inside your cheek. Have the person squeeze a small amount of frosting into your mouth and massage the outside of your cheek.

3. Keep doing step 2 until the ambulance arrives.

Blood Glucose, Self-Tests

Self-tests are tests you do yourself. A blood glucose self-test tells you how much glucose is in your blood at any one time. Anyone with diabetes can benefit from self-tests.

WHY TEST?

When you found out you had diabetes, you and your health care team worked out a diabetes-care plan. The plan was set up to help you keep your blood glucose levels in your ideal range (see Blood Glucose). Your plan may include a diet, regular exercise, insulin, or diabetes pills.

One of the best ways to keep track of how well your plan is working is to test your blood glucose. Testing helps you find out what happens to your blood glucose level when you eat certain foods, do certain exercises, or lose weight. Testing helps you find out what happens to your blood glucose level when you take insulin or diabetes pills, are sick, or are under stress.

A blood test can help you decide how to take care of your diabetes. Tests may prompt you to eat a snack, take more insulin, or exercise more. Tests may alert you to treat high or low blood glucose.

HOW TO TEST

You test your blood glucose with either a glucose meter or test strips that you read by eye. It's important to follow the instructions that come with the product you buy.

Most glucose self-tests go like this:

1. Wash your hands in warm, soapy water. Dry them.

2. Prick your finger with a lancet.

3. Let a drop of blood fall on a test strip pad.

4. Wait.

5. Read your blood glucose number in the window on the meter or match the color of the strip to a color chart to find your glucose range.

WHEN TO TEST

Your doctor or diabetes educator can help you figure out when to test. Testing at specific times can be useful. For instance, a test done 1 or 2 hours after a meal lets you see how high your blood glucose rises after you eat certain kinds and amounts of foods. A test at 2 or 3 AM tells you whether you have low blood glucose at night. There are eight test times for you to choose from:

1. Before breakfast

2. 1 to 2 hours after breakfast

3. Before lunch

4. 1 to 2 hours after lunch

5. Before supper

6. 1 to 2 hours after supper

7. Before bedtime

8. At 2 or 3 AM

The more you test, the more you will know about your blood glucose levels. The more you know about your blood glucose levels, the better able you will be to get those levels in your ideal range. Here are some sample test times you may want to talk about with your health care team.

If you have type 1 diabetes

Test before each meal and at bedtime every day OR 3 days a week.

If you have type 2 diabetes and you are on insulin

Test two to four times a day. Vary the times you test.

If you have type 2 diabetes and you are on diabetes pills

Test one or two times a day. If you test once a day, do it before you eat breakfast. If you test twice a day, test first when you get up in the morning. Vary the time of the second test.

If you have type 2 diabetes and treat with diet and exercise only

Test before you eat breakfast. Test 1 to 2 hours after a meal.

DO EXTRA TESTS

- When your team is trying to find the best dose of insulin or diabetes pills for you.
- When you change your exercise program or meal plan.
- When you start a new drug that can affect your glucose level.
- When you think your glucose is low or high.
- When you are sick.
- When you are pregnant.
- Before and after exercise. Test during exercise when you have been exercising for more than an hour.
- Before you drive.
- Before activities that take a lot of concentration.

KEEP RECORDS

Be sure to write down your test results, date, and time. Do this even if you have a meter with a memory. Your doctor or diabetes educator can tell you what else to record, such as

- the foods you eat and when you eat them.
- times that you miss meals or snacks.
- times that you eat large or small meals.
- times that you drink alcohol.

- how much alcohol you drink.
- how much you weigh.
- how much insulin you take and when.
- how many diabetes pills you take and when.
- when and how long you exercise.
- when and how you treat low or high blood glucose.
- when you are ill, injured, stressed, or have just had surgery.

Share your records with your health care team. Together, you can make needed changes in your diabetes-care plan. A better plan makes it easier for you to care for your diabetes.

Blood Vessel Disease

People with diabetes are more likely to develop blood vessel disease than people without diabetes. Blood vessel disease is also known as atherosclerosis or hardening of the arteries.

In atherosclerosis, large blood vessels become narrowed or blocked by a buildup of fat and cholesterol. This buildup of fat and cholesterol may slow or stop blood flow.

Slow blood flow can damage the heart (coronary artery disease), the brain (cerebrovascular disease), or the legs and feet (peripheral vascular disease).

Lack of blood flow to the heart can cause a heart attack. Lack of blood flow to the brain can cause a stroke (see Heart Attack, Stroke). Decreased blood flow to the legs and feet can lead to amputation (see Foot Care).

Blood vessel disease comes on slowly. Often, you will not notice any signs until the damage has been done. If you have any of these signs, seek medical care right away.

SIGNS OF CORONARY ARTERY DISEASE

- Chest pain (called angina)
- Shortness of breath
- Sweating
- Dizziness
- Nausea
- Swollen ankles

SIGNS OF CEREBROVASCULAR DISEASE

- Weakness or numbness in your face, an arm, or a leg
- Blurring or loss of sight
- Difficulty speaking or understanding speech
- Severe headache

SIGNS OF PERIPHERAL VASCULAR DISEASE

- Cramping or tightness in one or both legs while walking, known as intermittent claudication
- Cold feet
- Pain in the legs or feet while at rest
- Loss of hair on the feet
- Shiny skin
- Thickened toenails

Blood vessel disease may begin in childhood and continue throughout life. People with diabetes often get blood vessel disease at a younger age than people without diabetes.

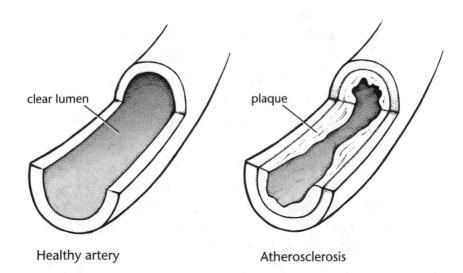

clear lumen   plaque

Healthy artery   Atherosclerosis

YOU ARE AT RISK FOR BLOOD VESSEL DISEASE IF

- You smoke.
- You have high blood pressure.
- You have high cholesterol levels.
- You are overweight.
- You have a family history of blood vessel disease.

Smoking narrows blood vessels. High blood pressure can weaken blood vessels. Narrow and weak blood vessels are more likely to get a buildup of fat and cholesterol.

High cholesterol means more cholesterol in the blood to stick to vessel walls. Being overweight causes your body to leave more fat in your blood.

TO REDUCE YOUR RISK OF BLOOD VESSEL DISEASE

- *Smoke less or quit.* Quitting can be hard but worth it. You can get support from a stop-smoking program or your health care team.
- *Control high blood pressure.* Many people can lower their blood pressure by losing weight through diet and exercise. Some people can lower blood pressure by cutting salt in their diet. For other people, blood pressure drugs are needed. If your doctor has prescribed blood pressure drugs, be sure to take them.
- *Nudge that cholesterol level down.* Try low-fat or reduced-fat versions of your favorite foods.
- *Exercise regularly.* Even a daily walk around the block helps. Find exercises you enjoy.
- *Aim for a healthy weight.* Combine an exercise program with a meal plan that suits your schedule and your tastes.
- *Get your diabetes under good control.* Test your blood glucose. Take your insulin or diabetes pills. Follow your meal plan. Stick with your exercise program. Keep records.

- ***Get regular medical checkups.*** Your doctor will check for blood vessel disease and help you keep tabs on your blood pressure, blood fat levels, and blood glucose control.

Complications

Complications are medical problems that occur more often in people with diabetes than in people without diabetes. Complications include eye diseases, kidney disease, nerve damage, and blood vessel disease (see each entry).

Your best defense against complications is keeping your blood glucose levels close to normal. Normal levels are the levels of people who do not have diabetes. The closer you can get to normal blood glucose levels, the more likely you are to prevent or delay complications. The Diabetes Control and Complications Trial proved it.

THE DIABETES CONTROL AND COMPLICATIONS TRIAL

The Diabetes Control and Complications Trial (DCCT) was a 10-year (1983–1993) medical study sponsored by the National Institutes of Health. It found that people with type 1 diabetes who kept their blood glucose levels close to normal had fewer complications than people whose blood glucose levels were higher.

Doctors studied complications in 1,441 people with type 1 diabetes. Some people used a standard therapy for their diabetes. Others used a more intensive therapy.

People on standard therapy took one or two insulin shots each day. Their insulin dose was kept about the same, and shots were taken at the same times each day. They tested their urine or blood for glucose. Most people on standard therapy had blood glucose levels above normal. But they did not have really high or low blood glucose levels.

People on intensive therapy took three or more insulin shots a day or used an insulin pump (see Insulin Pumps). They tested their blood glucose four or more times a day. They changed their insulin dose to fit the results of their blood glucose tests, how much they were going to eat, or what exercise they were going to do.

People on intensive therapy had blood glucose levels closer to normal. But they also had severe low blood glucose three times as often and gained more weight than people on the standard therapy.

WHAT THE DCCT MEANS FOR YOU

Talk with your doctor about what the results of this study mean for you. Maybe you want to try for tight control. Tight control is keeping your blood glucose levels close to normal. There is more than one way to gain tight control. You and your doctor can work out a plan for you whether you have type 1 or type 2 diabetes.

If you keep tight control of your blood glucose and still get a complication, it will most likely be milder and slower in coming. If you already have a complication, tight control can keep it from getting worse.

COPING WITH COMPLICATIONS

Learn all you can about your complication. The more you know about your complication, the more in control you will feel.

- *Talk with family and friends.* Tell them what's going on and what they can do to help.
- *Seek counseling.* If you find it hard to talk with family and friends, you may want to get counseling from a social worker or psychologist.
- *Join a support group.* Other people who have your complication can give you moral support. And you may get new ideas on treat-

ment options or doctors. Your doctor or local American Diabetes Association chapter may be able to help you find a support group.

- *See a specialist.* Think about going to a specialist who deals with your complication. Your own doctor may be able to refer you to one.

- *Ask questions about treatments.* What are the treatments? What are the side effects of the treatments? How much do these treatments cost? How often will I need treatments? How many patients with this problem have you treated? What has happened to those patients?

- *Try to get a second opinion.* Check your health insurance. It might cover a second opinion.

- *Look for organizations that focus on your complication.* Organizations like the National Kidney Foundation, the American Foundation for the Blind, and the National Amputation Foundation have programs and services. To find out more about them, look in The Encyclopedia of Associations. It's in most libraries.

- *Think positive.* Thinking good thoughts about yourself and about things in your life can make your life happier. Maybe even longer. Thinking too much about things you don't like or that make you angry or sad can only make living with complications harder for you and your loved ones.

Coping With Diabetes

Diabetes never goes away or even takes a vacation. It is a chronic disease that can be controlled but not cured. Living with diabetes is not only hard on your body but also hard on your mind.

You may at times deny that you have diabetes or feel angry or depressed about it. These feelings are normal. They may help you cope with having diabetes. They can be part of the process you go through before you accept diabetes.

Accepting diabetes means that you take responsibility for managing it, staying in good health, and living a full life. Accepting diabetes means you do not ignore diabetes and let it become a more serious health problem.

The best way to cope with diabetes is to accept it. But what if you get stuck in the process? If you are stuck in denial, anger, or depression for a long time, you may stop taking care of your diabetes.

DENIAL

Almost everybody goes through denial when they are first diagnosed with diabetes. The trouble comes when you keep on denying your diabetes. Continued denial keeps you from learning what you need to know to stay healthy. If you hear yourself thinking or saying some of these words, you may be denying some part of your diabetes care:

"One bite won't hurt."

"This sore will heal by itself."

"I'll go to the doctor later."

"I don't have time to do it."

"My diabetes isn't serious."

"I only take a pill, not shots."

"My insurance doesn't cover that."

Breaking away from denial

- Write down your diabetes-care plan and your health goals. Know why each part of your plan is important. Accept that it will take time to reach your goals.

- Talk to your diabetes educator about your diabetes-care plan. Together you may be able to come up with a better plan.

- Tell your friends and family how you take care of your diabetes. Tell them how they can help you.

ANGER

Anger is a powerful emotion. If you don't use anger, it will use you. To gain control over your anger, learn more about it. Start an anger diary. Write down when you felt angry, where you were, who you were with, why you felt angry, and what you did. After a few weeks, read it over. Try to understand your anger. What are you angry about? Usually under your anger are hurt feelings.

The better you understand your anger, the better you will be able to control it. How you use the energy of your anger is up to you. Plan to use your anger in a way that helps you next time.

How to control your anger

Defuse it. Talk slowly, take deep breaths, get a drink of water, sit down, lean back, keep your hands down at your sides.

Let it out. Do a physical activity like jogging or raking leaves. Cry over a sad movie. Write down on a piece of paper what you feel like saying or shouting.

Make it trivial. Ask yourself just how important it is. Some things are just too trivial to be worth your anger.

Laugh at it. Find something funny about it. Sometimes laughter can push out anger.

Let it give you strength. Anger can give you the courage to speak up for yourself or act to protect someone else.

DEPRESSION

Feeling down once in a while is normal. But feeling really sad and hopeless for 2 weeks or more might be a sign of serious depression.

You may be depressed if

- You no longer take interest or pleasure in things you used to enjoy doing.
- You have trouble falling asleep, wake often during the night, or want to sleep a lot more than usual.
- You wake up earlier than usual and cannot get back to sleep.
- You eat more or less than you used to. You quickly gain or lose weight.
- You have trouble concentrating. Other thoughts or feelings distract you.
- You have no energy. You feel tired all the time.
- You are so nervous or anxious, you can't sit still.
- You are less interested in sex.
- You cry often.
- You feel you never do anything right and are a burden to others.
- You feel sad or worse in the morning than you do the rest of the day.
- You feel you want to die or are thinking about ways to hurt yourself.

If you have three or more of these signs, get help. If you have one or two of these signs and have been feeling bad for 2 weeks or more, get help.

Help for depression

Talk to your doctor first. There may be a physical cause for your depression. If you and your doctor rule out physical causes, your doctor will likely refer you to a mental health professional. Treatment may involve counseling or antidepressant medication or both.

HOW TO COPE WITH DIABETES

Once you have made it through any denial, anger, or depression, you are on your way to accepting your diabetes. Accepting your diabetes is the way to cope with it.

Accept that diabetes care is up to you. You are the one who decides what to eat, how much to exercise, and when to test your blood glucose. Accept this for what it is—control. You are in control.

Learn as much about diabetes as you can. Your local chapter or affiliate of the American Diabetes Association can help. Read. Ask questions. Take diabetes education classes. Go to diabetes support groups.

Share what you have learned with your family and friends. The more they know, the better they will be able to help you. Tell them how you feel about diabetes.

Keep active in your hobbies, activities, and sports. You'll show everyone, including yourself, that you're still the same person. You can still have lots of fun.

Dental Care

Having diabetes puts you at risk for gum disease and other mouth infections. Infections can make your blood glucose level go up. And a high blood glucose level can make mouth infections even worse. You can protect yourself by knowing the signs of gum disease and other mouth infections and by knowing how to take care of your teeth.

GUM DISEASE

Gum disease is an infection of your gums. It starts with plaque. Plaque is a sticky film of germs that forms on your teeth. Plaque lives at your gum line. If you don't brush and floss your teeth to remove the plaque, it hardens into tartar. Tartar builds up under your gum line. Then more plaque forms over the tartar. Plaque and tartar irritate your gums. Your gums can become red, swollen, and tender. Then even gentle brushing can make your sore gums bleed. This is called gingivitis. If you ignore gingivitis, the gum disease can get worse.

As gum disease gets worse, your gums begin to pull away from your teeth. Part of your tooth's root may show or your teeth may look longer. Pockets form between your teeth and gums. These pockets fill with germs and pus. This is called periodontitis.

When this happens, you may need surgery to save your teeth. If nothing is done, the disease can destroy your jaw bone. Your teeth may start to move or get loose. They may

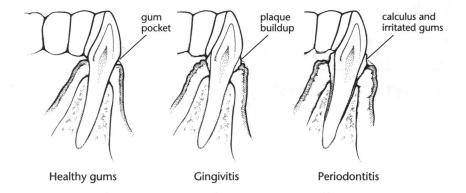

Healthy gums   Gingivitis   Periodontitis

fall out or have to be pulled. Know the warning signs of gum disease so you don't let it get this far.

Signs of gum disease

- Red gums
- Swollen or tender gums
- Gums that bleed when you brush or floss
- Gums that have pulled away from your teeth
- Pus between your teeth and gums when you press on the gums
- Bad breath
- Loose teeth
- Teeth that are moving away from each other
- A change in the way your teeth fit when you bite
- A change in the way your partial dentures fit

See your dentist if you have any of these signs.

OTHER MOUTH INFECTIONS

Mouth infections affect small areas in your mouth rather than your whole mouth. They can be caused by germs or a fungus. Know the warning signs of mouth infections.

Signs of mouth infections

- Swelling around your teeth or gums or anywhere in your mouth
- Pus around your teeth or gums or anywhere in your mouth
- White or red patches anywhere in your mouth
- Pain in your mouth or sinuses that does not go away
- Dark spots or holes on your teeth
- Teeth that hurt when you eat something cold, hot, or sweet
- Pain when chewing

See your dentist if you have any of these signs.

TO PROTECT YOUR TEETH

Control your blood glucose. If you keep your blood glucose at healthy levels, you'll lower your risk of gum disease and other mouth infections.

Keep your teeth clean. Brush your teeth with a fluoride toothpaste at least twice a day. Better yet, brush after every meal. Be careful not to brush too hard. You may wear away your gums. A soft toothbrush with rounded or polished bristles is easiest on your gums. Be sure to replace your toothbrush every 3 or 4 months, or sooner if the bristles are worn.

Floss your teeth at least once a day. If you don't like to use floss, try interdental picks or sticks. Flossing or picking cleans plaque and bits of food from between your teeth. Brushing removes plaque and bits of food from the surfaces of your teeth.

Go to your dentist. Have your dentist or dental hygienist clean your teeth every 6 months. These cleanings get rid of plaque and tartar. Make sure your dentist takes full mouth X rays every 2 years to check for bone loss. Some people show no other signs of periodontitis. Let your dentist know you have diabetes.

Diet

The healthiest diet or meal plan is low in saturated fat and cholesterol, has a moderate amount of protein, and is high in complex carbohydrates and fiber. This kind of diet can help protect you from heart disease, blood vessel disease, heart attack and stroke, colon and intestinal diseases, and some cancers.

LOW IN FAT AND CHOLESTEROL

For a low-fat, low-cholesterol diet, you'll want to eat fewer foods that have a lot of fat and cholesterol. When you do eat foods that are high in fat, choose foods that have more unsaturated fat. Saturated fats raise your cholesterol level more than anything else you eat. Unsaturated fats actually lower your cholesterol level.

Cholesterol is found in animal foods. Plant foods do not have cholesterol. Foods high in cholesterol include eggs, whole milk, regular cheeses, and meats.

Saturated fats are found in animal foods and some plant foods. Foods that have a lot of saturated fat include meat, whole-milk dairy products, lard, shortening, and coconut and palm oils.

Unsaturated fats are found in plant foods. Unsaturated fats can be polyunsaturated or monounsaturated. Vegetable oils, such as corn, cottonseed, safflower, soybean, and sunflower, are high in polyunsaturated fats. Oils that have mostly monounsaturated fats include olive, avocado, almond, canola, and peanut.

To cut fat and cholesterol

Dairy

- Use skim or 1% milk in place of whole or 2% milk, half and half, or cream.
- Use flavored low-fat or nonfat yogurt in place of flavored whole-milk yogurt.
- Use plain low-fat or nonfat yogurt in place of cream, sour cream, or mayonnaise.
- Use pureed low-fat or nonfat cottage cheese with a little lemon juice in place of sour cream.
- Use low-fat cream cheese or pureed low-fat cottage cheese in place of regular cream cheese.
- Use low-fat or nonfat cheeses in place of regular cheeses.
- Use frozen low-fat yogurt, fat-free ice cream, or sherbet in place of premium ice cream.

Eggs

- Limit whole eggs to three or four a week. You can use egg substitutes.
- In recipes, replace some of the whole eggs with egg whites. Two egg whites equal one whole egg.

Fats and oils

- Replace butter, regular margarine, lard, or shortening with soft tub, liquid, light, or diet margarine. You'll get less saturated fat.
- Replace butter or margarine with unsaturated oils. Try to cook food in a tablespoon or less of an unsaturated oil.
- Replace cooking oils with nonstick vegetable sprays, wine, or low-fat or nonfat broth.
- Replace regular oil-based salad dressings with low-fat or nonfat salad dressings. On salads, try lemon juice, or just salt and pepper, instead of dressing.

Meats

- Try to eat less meat. Keep your portion size to 3 ounces, about the size of a deck of cards.
- Choose lean cuts of meat rather than fatty cuts. Some lean cuts include top round steak, eye round roast, pork tenderloin, lamb shank, and veal leg.
- Use low-fat cooking methods, such as grilling or broiling, instead of frying.

Poultry

- Choose chicken and turkey breast.
- They have the least amount of fat. Don't eat the skin.

Fish

- Try to eat more fish. Most fish are naturally low in fat and calories. Fish oils have omega-3 fatty acids, which may protect you from heart disease.
- Steam, poach, or grill your fish.

MODERATE IN PROTEIN

For a diet that is moderate in protein, get your protein from foods that are low in fat, calories, and cholesterol.

Meats, poultry, eggs, milk, and cheese are high in protein. But they are also high in saturated fat and cholesterol. If you eat them, stick with lean cuts and low-fat versions.

A better choice for protein is fish and shellfish. Most fish and shellfish are lower in saturated fat and cholesterol than meat. You can also get protein from legumes (beans, peas, and lentils), grains, and vegetables. These are good choices for protein because they are low in fat and calories and have no cholesterol. Nuts and seeds have a good amount of protein in them, and most of the fat they contain is unsaturated.

HIGH IN COMPLEX CARBOHYDRATES AND FIBER

For a high-carbohydrate, high-fiber diet, choose fruits, vegetables, legumes, and grains. All are low in fat and have no cholesterol.

HIGH-FIBER FOODS

Fruits	Vegetables	Legumes	Grains
Apples	Bamboo shoots	Black beans	Barley
Blackberries		Chickpeas	Buckwheat
Blueberries	Broccoli	Cowpeas	Bulgur wheat
Dates	Brussels sprouts	Green peas	
Figs	Cabbage	Kidney beans	Corn bran
Oranges	Carrots		Cornmeal
Peaches	Corn	Lentils	Oat bran
Pears	Parsnips	Lima beans	Oatmeal
Prunes	Spinach	Navy beans	Rice bran
Raisins	Squash	Northern beans	Rye
Raspberries	Sweet potatoes	Pinto beans	Wheat bran
Strawberries		Soybeans	Wheat germ
Artichoke hearts	Yams	Split peas	Whole wheat

Dietitian

A dietitian is an expert in food and nutrition. Food is a key part of your diabetes care. A dietitian can help you figure out your food needs based on your weight, lifestyle, diabetes pills or insulin, other drugs you may be taking, and your health goals. Dietitians can teach you many useful skills, such as how to

- Make a meal plan.
- Use a meal plan.
- Read food labels.
- Choose wisely when grocery shopping.
- Choose wisely from restaurant menus.
- Turn a fatty recipe into a low-fat one.
- Find cookbooks and food guides.
- Find out how the foods you eat affect your blood fat levels.
- Find out how the foods you eat affect your blood glucose levels.
- Treat yourself for low blood glucose.

When your weight, lifestyle, medical needs, or health goals change, your food needs are likely to change, too. Your dietitian can help you adjust your meal plan to those changes.

The American Diabetes Association recommends that all adults with diabetes see a dietitian every 6 months to a year.

WHEN YOU LOOK FOR A DIETITIAN

Look for the initials RD after a dietitian's name. RD stands for registered dietitian. A registered dietitian has met standards set by the American Dietetic Association. An RD may also have a master's degree.

You might see the initials LD after a dietitian's name. LD stands for licensed dietitian. Many states require dietitians to have a license.

Look for a dietitian who has worked with people who have diabetes. The letters CDE after a dietitian's name mean that he or she is trained and up-to-date in diabetes care and treatment. CDE stands for Certified Diabetes Educator.

Your doctor or local area hospitals may be able to recommend a dietitian. Or The American Dietetic Association Consumer Nutrition Hot Line at 1-800-366-1655 can refer you to a dietitian.

Doctor

Your diabetes doctor may be an endocrinologist or a diabetologist. An endocrinologist is a medical doctor who has special training and certification in treating diseases such as diabetes. A diabetologist is a medical doctor who has an interest in diabetes. Your diabetes doctor may be an internist, a family practitioner, or a general practitioner who cares for people with diabetes.

The kind of diabetes doctor you go to is not as important as the kind of care you get. The American Diabetes Association has guidelines to let your doctor know how to care for you. These guidelines are called "Standards of Medical Care for Patients With Diabetes Mellitus." They can be found in the *Clinical Practice Recommendations* yearly supplement to the January issue of the journal *Diabetes Care*. Be sure to let your doctor know about them.

The guidelines can help you, too. They let you know what to expect from your doctor. That way, you can check whether your doctor is giving you the best care. Here's a sample of what the guidelines cover.

FIRST VISIT

During your first visit to a new doctor who will treat your diabetes, ask the doctor to help you put together a health care team. A health care team can help you make a plan to care for your diabetes. A diabetes-care plan will tell you what you need to know about food, exercise, diabetes pills or insulin, and blood glucose testing.

At your first visit, your doctor or health care team member will

- Ask when you found out you had diabetes.
- Ask for results of those lab tests.
- Ask who else in your family has diabetes.
- Ask how you treat your diabetes.
- Ask what and when you eat.
- Ask how often and how hard you exercise.
- Ask about your weight.
- Ask if you smoke.
- Ask if you have high blood pressure.
- Ask if you have high cholesterol.
- Ask if you have had ketones in your urine.
- Ask if you have had low blood glucose.
- Ask what infections you have had.
- Ask what complications you have had.
- Ask what treatments you have been given.
- Ask what drugs you are taking.
- Ask what other medical problems you have had.
- Ask if you had problems when pregnant.
- Measure your height, weight, and blood pressure.
- Look in your eyes and ask about eye problems.
- Look in your mouth and ask about dental problems.
- Feel your neck to check your thyroid gland and do tests if needed.
- Listen to your heart through a stethoscope.
- Feel your abdomen to check your liver and other organs.
- Look at your hands and fingers.
- Look at your bare feet.
- Check the sensation and pulses in your feet.
- Check your skin.

- Test your reflexes.
- Take your pulse.
- Request blood and urine samples for tests.

FUTURE VISITS

Your doctor will tell you when to come for another checkup. Your doctor may want to see you two or three times a year.

If you take insulin or if you have poor blood glucose control, your doctor may want to see you four or more times a year.

If you have complications or if you start something new in your care plan, your doctor may want to see you even more often.

When you return, expect your doctor or other members of your health care team to

- Ask to see your blood glucose records.
- Ask if your blood glucose has been too high or too low.
- Ask about signs that might mean you are getting a complication.
- Ask if you have been sick since your last visit.
- Ask what drugs you are taking now.
- Ask if your life has changed.
- Ask if you have had problems with your plan.
- Weigh you and take your blood pressure.
- Look in your eyes.
- Look at your bare feet.
- Request blood for a glycohemoglobin test.
- Request a urine test.
- Request tests of kidney function.
- Request tests of blood fat levels.
- Go over your plan to see if you have met your goals.
- Discuss changes in your plan if you both agree that changes are needed.

Eating Disorders

Two eating disorders—anorexia and bulimia—may be more common in people with diabetes than in people without diabetes. Researchers are not sure why this is so, but both diabetes and eating disorders have in common a focus on food, diet, and weight.

ANOREXIA

People with anorexia have an intense fear of becoming fat. To stay thin, they starve themselves. They may have secretive or strange eating habits, such as cutting food into tiny pieces. They may refuse to eat with other people. To lose more weight, they may exercise very hard. People with anorexia see themselves as fat even when they are very thin.

BULIMIA

People with bulimia are overly concerned with their body shape and weight. They will binge and purge twice a week or more to prevent weight gain. Bingeing is eating a large amount of food (often several thousand calories worth) at one time.

During a binge, people with bulimia feel out of control and frightened. After a binge, they feel depressed and have low self-esteem. They purge themselves by making themselves throw up or by taking laxatives or diuretics to cause diarrhea. They may also try to purge themselves by strict dieting or fasting, or by exercising very hard. People with bulimia may be overweight, underweight, or of normal weight.

EATING DISORDERS AND DIABETES CONTROL

Most people with diabetes who have an eating disorder have poor diabetes control. A few manage to keep their diabetes in good control. Those with bulimia take more insulin after a binge. Those with anorexia lower their insulin dose to match their lower food intake. Others just work hard to keep their eating disorder under control so that they do not upset their diabetes control.

EATING DISORDERS AND WEIGHT CONTROL

An eating disorder makes weight control very difficult. People with diabetes who have an eating disorder may reduce or omit their insulin dose to lose weight. Many people who try this are overweight. Others are of normal weight or even low weight.

Stopping insulin causes a dangerous kind of weight loss. The body loses water weight and can become dehydrated. Without enough insulin, the body does not get enough blood glucose for energy. The body uses up its stores of glycogen in the liver. Then it starts to break down fat tissues, muscles, and body organs. If insulin is not resumed, the person eventually dies.

EATING DISORDERS AND HEALTH

People with eating disorders are more likely to have digestion problems, heart problems, and other problems brought on by starvation, self-induced vomiting, and abuse of laxatives and diuretics. In addition, people with diabetes who have an eating disorder are more likely to get

- High ketones
- High blood glucose
- Low blood glucose
- Eye disease

- Kidney disease
- Nerve disease

HELP FOR EATING DISORDERS

A person with an eating disorder needs the help of a physician, mental health professional, and dietitian. Ask a family doctor or counselor for a referral. Some clinics and health care centers specialize in treating people with eating disorders. Check the white pages of a phone book under "Eating Disorders."

Most eating disorders can be treated with outpatient psychotherapy or behavioral therapy and family or group therapy. Drugs for depression are sometimes used. If a person with an eating disorder refuses help and his or her life is in danger, he or she may be admitted to the psychiatric unit of a hospital for treatment.

Employment Rights

People who have diabetes are more likely to have a hard time finding jobs than people who do not have diabetes. And they lose jobs more easily. This happens because some employers are afraid to hire people who have diabetes. They worry that diabetes will interfere with the job. Or that it will make health insurance premiums higher for the company.

You don't have to tell an employer that you have diabetes. An employer cannot ask you about your health or make you get a physical examination before offering you a job. However, some jobs require you to get a physical examination after you are hired.

After you are hired, you may want to tell your employer about your diabetes. Telling your employer about your diabetes is the only way your employment rights will be protected by The Americans With Disabilities Act of 1990.

The Americans With Disabilities Act is a civil rights law. Title I of this law protects the employment rights of people with diabetes who are considered disabled.

YOU ARE CONSIDERED DISABLED IF ONE OF THESE STATEMENTS IS TRUE:

1. Diabetes greatly limits one or more of your major life activities. Major life activities include seeing, hearing, speaking, walking, breathing, doing manual tasks, learning, caring for yourself, and working.

2. At one time, diabetes greatly limited one or more of your major life activities.

3. Your employer sees you as disabled because you have diabetes. It does not matter if your diabetes is well controlled.

YOU ARE PROTECTED BY THE AMERICANS WITH DISABILITIES ACT WHEN

- You apply for a job.
- You are hired.
- You are trained.
- You are paid.
- You are given benefits.
- You are promoted.
- You are granted tenure.
- You take a leave of absence.
- You are laid off.
- You are fired.
- Your employer recruits people for a job.
- Your employer advertises for a job.

Your spouse, parents, roommates, and friends are also protected by The Americans With Disabilities Act if they are discriminated against (treated unfairly) because you have diabetes.

The Americans With Disabilities Act applies to private companies, state and local governments, employment agencies, and labor unions.

The Act does not apply to employers with fewer than 15 workers, Native American tribes, tax-exempt private clubs, and the federal government. People who work for the federal government or for organizations that get federal funds are protected by the Federal Rehabilitation Act of 1973.

If neither Act protects you, check with your state and city. They may have their own employment rights laws.

Job discrimination can be hard to prove. If you think an employer has discriminated against you because of diabetes, follow these steps:

1. Try to solve the problem by talking directly with the employer.

2. Get the help of a union or employee group.

3. Think about seeing a lawyer. With a telephone call or letter, a lawyer may be able to resolve the problem easily.

4. File charges with the Equal Employment Opportunity Commission. Look up their number in the blue pages of the phone book under U.S. Government.

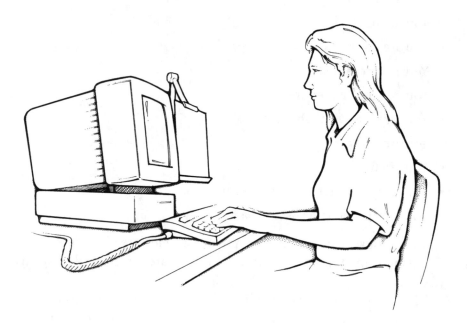

Exercise, Aerobic

Aerobic exercises are ones that use your heart, lungs, arms, and legs. By working these parts of your body, you can improve your blood flow, reduce your risk of heart disease, and lower your blood pressure. You can also lower your LDL cholesterol and triglycerides and raise your HDL cholesterol (the good kind).

When you do aerobic exercises, you breathe harder and your heart beats faster. This builds your endurance and increases your energy. You may find that aerobic exercise helps you sleep better, makes you feel less stressed, balances your emotions, and improves your sense of well-being.

Aerobic exercise is not only good for your health but is also good for your diabetes. Aerobic exercise makes your insulin work harder and faster, reduces your body fat, and helps you lose weight. If you don't exercise already, your doctor may advise you to start.

WHAT TO DO BEFORE YOU START

Check with your doctor before you start any exercise. Your doctor may want to run some tests to see how your heart, blood vessels, eyes, feet, and nerves are doing. Your blood pressure, blood fat levels, glycohemoglobin levels, and body fat might also be checked. Your doctor or nurse can tell you how to adjust your diabetes-care plan for exercise.

WHAT AEROBIC EXERCISES TO DO

Some exercises may make heart, eye, feet, or nerve problems worse. Find out from your doctor what kinds of exercises are safe for you to do. Pick from these exercises a few you think you might enjoy. Then learn the right way to do each exercise. Here are some examples of aerobic exercises:

- Aerobics classes or videotapes
- Bicycling
- Dancing
- Jogging
- Jumping rope
- Rowing
- Running
- Skating (roller, ice, in-line)
- Skiing (downhill, cross-country)
- Stair climbing
- Swimming
- Walking
- Water exercises

HOW LONG AND HOW OFTEN TO EXERCISE

If you are just starting to exercise after a long time of little or no activity, go for 5 minutes. Build up to short bouts of exercise that add up to at least 30 minutes a day. For example, you might try brisk walking or stair climbing for 10 minutes three times a day or for 15 minutes twice a day.

Exercising for less than 15 minutes a day is not likely to improve your health. Gradually build up to 20 to 60 minutes of continuous aerobic exercise three to five times a week. The 20 to 60 minutes of aerobic exercise does not include your warm-up and cooldown.

A warm-up will slowly raise your heart rate, warm your muscles, and help prevent injuries. A cooldown will lower your heart rate and slow your breathing. Warm up for 5 to 10 minutes before aerobic exercise, and cool down for 5 to 10 minutes after aerobic exercise. As a warm-up or a cooldown, you could gently stretch, walk, or slowly bicycle.

HOW HARD TO EXERCISE

Your doctor, nurse, or exercise specialist can tell you how hard to exercise by giving you a number. The number is a percentage. It may be as low as 40 percent or as high as 70 percent. It is a percentage of your capacity for exercise (your maximum aerobic capacity). There are a few ways to figure out your maximum aerobic capacity. Here's one easy way.

Subtract your age from 220. The answer is your maximum heart rate. For example, if you are 40, your maximum heart rate is 180. To exercise at 60 percent of your maximum aerobic capacity, keep your pulse at 108 beats per minute ($180 \times 60\% = 108$). A nurse can show you how to take your pulse.

If you have nerve damage or take certain blood pressure drugs, your heart may beat more slowly. Check with your doctor about this. If your heart does beat more slowly, your heart rate is not a good guide for how hard to exercise. Instead, exercise at what you feel is a moderate level of exertion. Moderate is not too hard and not too easy. You should be able to talk while you're exercising.

Signs that you are exercising too hard

- You can't talk while exercising.
- Your pulse is higher than the pulse you are trying to maintain.
- You rate your level of exertion as hard or very hard.

WHEN TO TEST YOUR BLOOD GLUCOSE

Exercise usually makes your blood glucose level go down. But if your blood glucose level is high before you start, exercise can make it go up even higher.

If you take insulin or diabetes pills, exercise can make your blood glucose level go too low. The best way to find out how exercise affects your blood glucose is to test before and after exercising.

Test your blood glucose twice before exercise. Test at 30 minutes before exercise and again just before you begin. This tells you whether your blood glucose level is rising, stable, or dropping. If it is rising, wait until it is stable. If it is dropping, you may need an extra snack to get it stable. When it is stable, begin your exercise.

Be ready to test your blood glucose during exercise. There are times during exercise that you may want to stop and check your blood glucose:

- When you are trying an exercise for the first time and want to see how it is affecting your blood glucose.
- When you feel your blood glucose might be going too low.
- When you will be exercising for more than 1 hour (test every 30 minutes).

Test your blood glucose after exercise. When you exercise, your body uses glucose that is stored in your muscles and liver. After exercise, your body restores glucose to your muscles and liver by removing it from your blood. This can go on for as long as 10 to 24 hours. During this time, blood glucose levels may fall too low.

WHEN TO EAT SNACKS

Depending on how hard and how long you exercise, you may need to eat extra snacks. A snack can be a piece of fruit, half a cup of juice, half a bagel, or a small roll. Talk with your dietitian about what snacks are good for you and when it is best for you to eat them. If you take insulin or diabetes pills, you may need to eat a snack before, during, or after exercise.

If your blood glucose level is less than 100 mg/dl before exercise
  You may need to eat a snack before you start.

If your blood glucose level is between 100 and 250 mg/dl before exercise AND you will be exercising for more than 1 hour
  You will need to eat snacks every 30 minutes to 1 hour.

If your blood glucose level is between 100 and 250 mg/dl before exercise AND you will be exercising for less than 1 hour
  You probably will not need to eat a snack.

WHEN AND WHAT TO DRINK

Exercise makes you sweat. Sweating means you are losing fluid. To replace lost fluids, be sure to drink after exercise or during exercise, if the exercise is intense.

Water is usually the best choice. But if you are exercising for a long time, you may want a drink that contains carbohydrate. Choose drinks that are no more than 10 percent carbohydrate, such as sports drinks or diluted fruit juices (1/2 cup fruit juice, 1/2 cup water).

WHEN TO EXERCISE

A good time to exercise is 1 to 3 hours after you finish a meal or snack. The food you have eaten will help keep your blood glucose level from falling too low.

DO NOT EXERCISE WHEN

- Your blood glucose level is over 300 mg/dl.
- Your insulin or diabetes pills are peaking.
- You have ketones in your urine.
- You have numbness, tingling, or pain in your feet or legs.
- You are short of breath.
- You are ill.

- You have a serious injury.
- You feel dizzy.
- You feel sick to your stomach.
- You have pain/tightness in your chest, neck, shoulders, or jaw.
- You have blurred sight or blind spots.

Exercise, Flexibility

Flexibility is how far you can stretch the muscles around your joints without stiffness, resistance, or pain. Flexible muscles and joints are less likely to get injured when you use them.

One of the best ways to become more flexible is to stretch every day. Stretch a little bit throughout the day to relieve muscle tension and stress. Make stretching a part of your workout.

There are lots of different stretches. You can find them in books, on videos, and in exercise classes. Here are a few stretches for you to try. But first, some rules.

STRETCHING RULES

- Go slowly and smoothly.
- Remember to breathe.
- Don't bounce.
- Relax any tension you feel.
- Go only as far as you can without pain.
- Hold for at least 8 to 10 seconds.

Calf stretch. Face a wall, about a foot away. Stand with one foot in front of the other, toes straight ahead. Keep both feet flat on the floor. Bend your front knee. Slowly lean forward, and rest your forearms on the wall. Press your rear heel into the floor. Repeat with your other leg.

Quadriceps (front of thigh) stretch. Stand with legs straight or slightly bent. Bend one leg back, lifting your foot off the floor. Grab the ankle of the bent leg with one hand. You may want to hold on to something for balance. Gently pull your foot up so your heel is headed for your bottom and hold. Release. Repeat with your other leg.

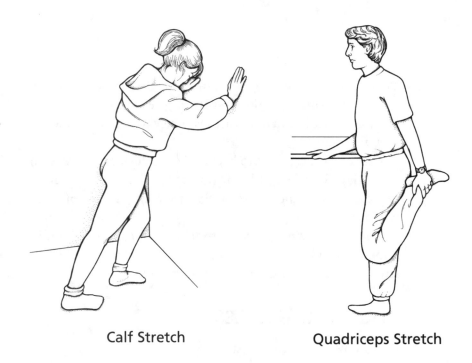

Calf Stretch   Quadriceps Stretch

Hamstrings (back of thigh) stretch. Lie on your back. Bend your legs, feet on the floor. Lift one leg up. Keep it slightly bent. Grasp the leg at the calf with both hands. Holding on to your leg, try to straighten it. Release. Straighten again and release. Repeat with your other leg.

Back and hips stretch. Sit with one leg straight out. Bend your other leg. Cross your bent leg over your straight leg, placing the foot of your bent leg on the floor next to the knee of the straight leg. Breathe. Slowly twist your upper body in the direction of your straight leg. Keep turning your head to look behind you. Keep your shoulders relaxed and your chin level. Brace yourself by placing the elbow of the arm nearest your bent knee on the inside of your bent knee. Slowly unwind and rest both legs on the floor. Repeat on the other side.

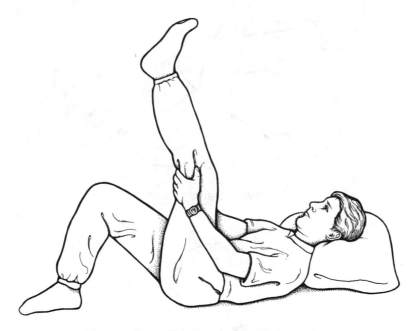

Hamstrings (back of thigh) Stretch

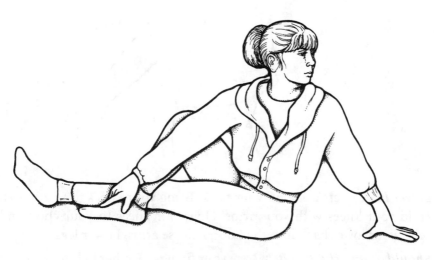

Back and Hips Stretch

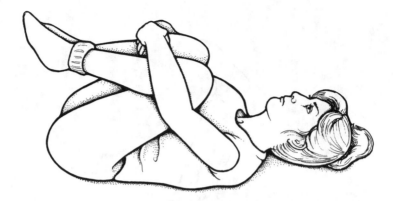

Lower Back Stretch

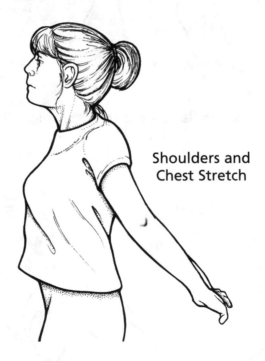

Shoulders and
Chest Stretch

Lower back stretch. Lie on your back. Bring your knees to your chest. Hold your knees with your arms. Hug your knees to your chest and press your lower back into the floor. Release arms. Lower legs.

Shoulders and chest stretch. Lace your fingers together behind you. Lift your arms up. Hold. Breathe. Slowly lower, and let go.

Arms stretch. Raise your arms over your head. Lace your fingers together with palms up. Press your arms upward.

Neck stretch. Center your head over your shoulders. Look down. Let your head roll toward your chest. Bring your head back to the center. Look up. Point your chin toward the ceiling. Bring your head back to the center. Look over one shoulder. Bring your head back to the center. Look over the other shoulder. Repeat slowly.

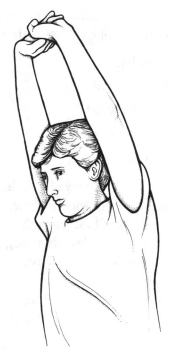

Arms Stretch

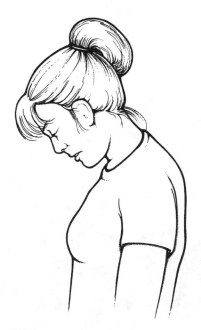

Neck Stretch 1

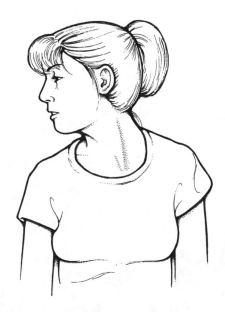

Neck Stretch 2

If you would like more of a challenge for your muscles and joints, consider one of these other flexibility exercises:

- Ballet
- Gymnastics
- Martial arts
- Modern dance
- Yoga

Before you try any of these flexibility exercises, check with your doctor. Some of the movements may not be safe for you.

You can best learn the flexibility exercises from an instructor. Many places offer classes for beginners. Community recreation centers often have classes at low cost.

If you are thinking of taking a class, you may want to watch at least one class before signing up. You might also want to ask if the teacher has experience teaching people with diabetes.

Exercise, Strength

Strength exercises are ones that work your muscles against a weight. Strength exercises include using weight machines, lifting free weights, doing calisthenics, and doing circuit training.

WEIGHT MACHINES

Weight machines allow you to change how much weight you want to lift by either placing a pin in a stack of weights or turning a valve that controls fluid pressure. Some well-known brands of weight machines are Nautilus, Universal, and Cybex.

FREE WEIGHTS

Free weights are not attached to another piece of equipment. Free weights include dumbbells and barbells. A dumbbell is a short bar you can lift with one hand. A barbell is a long bar you lift with both hands.

CALISTHENICS

In calisthenics, the weight you use is your own body. Calisthenics include push-ups, chin-ups, sit-ups, leg lifts, and squats. You can make your muscles work harder by strapping weights to your wrists or ankles or by using elastic bands.

CIRCUIT TRAINING

In circuit training, you go through a series of stations. At each station, you do a different exercise. You might use a weight machine, lift free weights, do an aerobic exercise, or do calisthenics. After you finish the exercise at one station, you have a short rest period before you go on to the next station.

WHY DO STRENGTH EXERCISES?

Strength exercises make your muscles stronger and more flexible and your bones sturdier. Strong muscles and bones are less likely to become injured. The stronger you are, the easier everyday physical tasks become, and the longer you can stay active without tiring.

WHAT TO DO BEFORE YOU START

See your doctor. Talk to your doctor before you start strength exercises. Some exercises may be better for you than others. Some may not be safe for you at all.

Choose your exercises. When you know the kinds of strength exercises that are safe for you, pick out 8 to 10 different ones. Be sure to pick ones that will work your legs and hips, chest, back, shoulders, arms, and abdomen. The idea is to work all your muscle groups. Your doctor may be able to help you choose them.

Learn how to do your exercises. Once you have chosen your exercises, learn the right way to do them. If you do exercises the wrong way, you might injure yourself. If the exercises you have chosen require you to use equipment that is new to you, learn how to use and adjust it. Find out how to use any safety equipment that goes along with your exercise, too.

HOW TO STRENGTHEN WITH WEIGHTS OR CALISTHENICS

As with any other exercise, warm up for 5 to 10 minutes before you begin, and cool down for 5 to 10 minutes after you finish. Try gentle stretching and slow walking or bicycling.

After you warm up, start with just 1 set of each exercise. A set is the number of times you repeat an exercise before you rest. Have an exercise specialist help you figure out how many repetitions to do of each exercise. Here are some general guidelines:

If the strength exercise is easy for you
Do it 15 to 20 times. Rest for 1 minute or less between sets.

If the strength exercise is moderate for you
Do it 8 to 12 times. Rest for 1 or 2 minutes between sets.

If the strength exercise is hard for you
Do it 2 to 6 times. Rest for 3 to 5 minutes between sets.

Remember, start with just 1 set. As you become stronger, you will be able to do more sets. Work your way up a little bit at a time to 2 or 3 sets of each exercise. Once you are doing 2 or 3 sets easily, you are ready to make the exercise harder by adding more weight.

Another thing to remember is to move your muscles through their full range of motion. This increases flexibility. A muscle that moves only part of the way loses flexibility. And keep breathing! Breathe in as you lower. Breathe out as you lift. If you don't like this pattern, then just breathe normally.

HOW LONG AND HOW OFTEN TO EXERCISE

Do your strength exercises for 20 to 30 minutes two or three times a week. Allow at least 1 day of rest between days you do the same strength exercises. To grow stronger, muscles need rest as well as exercise.

Eye Diseases

People with diabetes are more likely to get an eye disease than people without diabetes. The three main eye diseases that people with diabetes get are retinopathy, cataracts, and glaucoma. Of the three, retinopathy is the most common.

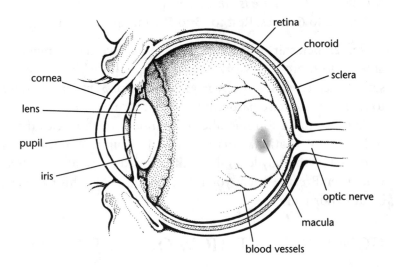

RETINOPATHY

The retina is the lining at the back of the eye that senses light. Small blood vessels bring oxygen to the retina. Retinopathy damages the small blood vessels in the retina. The two major types of retinopathy are called nonproliferative and proliferative.

Nonproliferative retinopathy

In nonproliferative (or background) retinopathy, the small blood vessels in the retina bulge and form pouches. This weakens the blood vessels. They may leak a bit of fluid. This leaking does not usually harm your sight. And, often, the disease never gets worse.

If the disease does get worse, the weak blood vessels leak a larger amount of fluid. They also leak blood and fats. This causes the retina to swell. The swelling will usually not harm your sight, unless it occurs in the center of the retina.

The center of the retina is called the macula. The macula lets you see fine details. Swelling in the macula is called macular edema. Macular edema can blur, distort, reduce, or darken your sight.

Proliferative retinopathy

Nonproliferative retinopathy may progress to proliferative retinopathy. In proliferative retinopathy, the small blood vessels are so damaged that they close off. In response, many new blood vessels grow in the retina. As these new blood vessels grow, they branch out to other parts of your eye.

These changes may not affect your sight. Or, these changes will make you less able to see things out of the sides of your eyes. You might also find it harder to see in the dark and to adjust from light to dark.

The new blood vessels are weak and can cause problems. They may break and bleed into the clear gel that fills the center of the eye. This is known as a vitreous hemorrhage. The most common signs of vitreous hemorrhage are blurring and floating spots. Vitreous hemorrhage can cause you to lose sight, if not treated.

The new blood vessels may cause scar tissue to grow on the retina. Scar tissue can wrinkle the retina and pull it out of place. A retina that has been pulled away from the back of the eye is called a detached retina. A detached retina will cause you to see a shadow or large dark area. It can endanger your sight.

Signs of retinopathy

- Your sight gets blurry.
- You see floating spots.
- You see a shadow or dark area.
- You can't see things out of the sides of your eyes.
- You have trouble seeing at night.
- You have trouble reading.
- Straight lines do not look straight.

If you have any of these signs, go to your eye doctor right away.

Special note: Usually, you can't see (or feel) the early signs of damage to your retina, but your eye doctor can. Be sure to have your eyes checked for retinopathy every year.

CATARACTS

A cataract clouds the eye's lens. The eye's lens is usually clear. The lens lies behind the iris (the colored part of your eye) and the pupil (the dark opening). The lens focuses light onto the retina. Clouding of the lens blocks light from entering.

Cataracts usually start out small. Some of them never worsen your sight. Others block most or all of your sight. How a cataract will affect your sight depends on three things: 1) how large or small it is, 2) how thin or thick it is, and 3) where it is on the lens.

Because of these three things, signs that you have a cataract may vary.

Signs of a cataract

- Your sight is hazy, fuzzy, or blurry.
- You think you need new glasses.
- Your new glasses don't help you see any better.
- You find it harder to read and do other close work.

- You blink a lot to see better.
- You feel you have a film over your eyes.
- You feel you are looking through a cloudy piece of glass, veils, or a waterfall.
- Light from the sun or a lamp seems too bright.
- At night, headlights on other cars cause more glare than before or look double or dazzling.
- Your pupil, which is usually black, looks gray, yellow, or white.
- Colors look dull.

If you have any of these signs, see your eye doctor.

GLAUCOMA

Glaucoma is a buildup of fluid in the eye. The fluid buildup causes increased pressure. The pressure can damage your optic nerve. Your optic nerve tells your brain what your eye sees. There are two kinds of glaucoma.

The most common type is chronic open-angle glaucoma. In this type, fluid pressure rises slowly over many years. You usually won't notice it. You might feel the increased pressure in your eye or your eyes may keep tearing.

As the glaucoma worsens, you may notice that your sight is slightly blurry or foggy. You may feel that your glasses should be changed. You may have a hard time seeing in the dark. If not treated, you may lose your sight.

The less common type of glaucoma is acute angle-closure glaucoma. In this type, fluid pressure builds up quickly. Your eyes hurt a lot. They are blurry and keep tearing. You see colored halos around bright lights. You may even vomit. *If you have any of these signs, go to a hospital emergency room right away.*

TO KEEP YOUR EYES FREE OF DISEASE

Keep your blood glucose levels close to normal. Keeping your blood glucose levels close to normal lowers your risk of getting eye diseases and slows down those that have started.

Control high blood pressure. High blood pressure can make eye diseases worse. You may be able to bring blood pressure down by losing weight, eating less salt, and avoiding alcohol. Your doctor can tell you about drugs to lower blood pressure.

Quit smoking. Smoking damages your blood vessels.

Lower high cholesterol. High cholesterol can also damage your blood vessels.

Get yearly eye exams by an eye doctor. Many eye diseases can do damage without causing signs you can see. An eye doctor has the tools and tests to find damage early. The earlier damage is found, the greater the chance that treatments can save your sight.

Food Labeling

Food labels now tell you almost everything you need to know about foods. The more you know about foods, the better food choices you can make, and the better you can control your diabetes.

One of the first things you might see on a food package is a nutrient claim, such as "reduced fat" or "low calorie." These claims have standard meanings. Some of these terms and their meanings are listed at the end of this section. But the most useful information on a food package is found in the Nutrition Facts box.

SERVING SIZES

Serving sizes are now more uniform in all brands of similar foods. In this way, you can more easily make comparisons. And the serving sizes are closer to the amounts people really eat. Serving sizes are given in both household (e.g., cup) and metric (e.g., gram) measures.

LIST OF NUTRIENTS

Nutrition Facts must list calories, calories from fat, total fat, saturated fat, cholesterol, sodium, total carbohydrate, dietary fiber, sugars, and protein. Nutrients that may also be listed include calories from saturated fat, polyunsaturated fat, monounsaturated fat, and potassium.

Nutrients listed are followed by a number. This number is the amount of that nutrient (in grams or milligrams) in one serving of the food.

Nutrition Facts

Serving Size 1 cup (228g)
Servings Per Container 2

Amount Per Serving

Calories 260   Calories from Fat 120

	% Daily Value*
Total Fat 13g	**20%**
Saturated Fat 5g	**25%**
Cholesterol 30mg	**10%**
Sodium 660mg	**28%**
Total Carbohydrate 31g	**10%**
Dietary Fiber 0g	**0%**
Sugars 5g	
Protein 5g	

Vitamin A 4%	•	Vitamin C 2%
Calcium 15%	•	Iron 4%

* Percent Daily Values are based on a 2,000 calorie diet. Your daily values may be higher or lower depending on your calorie needs:

		Calories:	2,000	2,500
Total Fat	Less than		65g	80g
Sat Fat	Less than		20g	25g
Cholesterol	Less than		300mg	300mg
Sodium	Less than		2,400mg	2,400mg
Total Carbohydrate			300g	375g
Dietary Fiber			25g	30g

Calories per gram:
Fat 9 • Carbohydrate 4 • Protein 4

BASIC FOOD LABEL
Source: Food and Drug Administration

VITAMINS AND MINERALS

Nutrition Facts must list the amounts of vitamin A, vitamin C, calcium, and iron. Other vitamins and minerals may also be listed. After the name of the vitamin or mineral is a number followed by a percent sign (%). This number is the percentage of the daily amount of the vitamin or mineral in one serving of the food. Higher numbers mean the food has more of that vitamin or mineral.

DAILY VALUES

Daily Values tell you how much of certain nutrients you need. Daily Values have been set for total fat, saturated fat, cholesterol, sodium, potassium, total carbohydrate, dietary fiber, and protein. There is no Daily Value for sugars because health experts have not agreed on the total amount of sugars a person should eat.

NUTRIENT CLAIMS

Term	Description
Calorie free	Less than 5 calories per serving
Cholesterol free	Less than 2 mg of cholesterol per serving and 2 g or less of saturated fat per serving
Fat free	Less than 0.5 g of fat per serving
Saturated fat free	Less than 0.5 g of saturated fat per serving
Sodium free	Less than 5 mg of sodium per serving
Sugar free	Less than 0.5 g of sugar per serving
Low calorie	40 calories or less per serving
Low cholesterol	20 mg or less of cholesterol per serving and 2 g or less of saturated fat per serving
Low fat	3 g or less of fat per serving
Low saturated fat	1 g or less of saturated fat per serving
Low sodium	140 mg or less of sodium per serving
Extra lean	Less than 5 g of fat, 2 g of saturated fat, and 95 mg of cholesterol per serving
Lean	Less than 10 g of fat, 4.5 g of saturated fat, and 95 mg of cholesterol per serving
Light or lite	33.3% fewer calories or 50% less fat per serving than comparison food
Reduced	25% less per serving than comparison food. Check label carefully. Some of these foods are still too high in fat and calories.

Daily Values are based on the number of calories you eat in a day. All packages with Nutrition Facts list Daily Values for people who eat 2,000 calories a day. Larger packages also list Daily Values for people who eat 2,500 calories a day.

Your own Daily Values may be higher or lower than those listed. The more calories you need to eat in a day, the higher your Daily Values. The fewer calories you need to eat in a day, the lower your Daily Values. With the help of a dietitian, you can figure out your own Daily Values to fit your calorie needs.

Percent Daily Values

Percent Daily Values tell you how much of the Daily Values of nutrients you use up when you eat one serving of the food. A higher percentage means you use up more of the Daily Value.

Foot Care

People with diabetes can get many kinds of foot problems. Even minor ones can turn into serious ones.

POOR CIRCULATION

Diabetes can narrow and harden the blood vessels in your feet (see Blood Vessel Disease). This can limit blood flow. A lack of blood to your feet can make them feel cold or look blue or puffy. Without enough blood, your feet may be less able to fight infection. Wounds may heal more slowly. Sometimes your wounds won't heal at all.

NERVE DAMAGE

Nerve damage can make your feet less able to feel pain, heat, and cold. That makes it easy to hurt your feet but hard to feel the hurt.

Nerve damage can affect the nerves that cause sweating. As a result, your feet may become dry and scaly. The skin may peel and crack.

Nerve damage can also deform your feet. Your toes may curl up. The ball of your foot may stick out more. Your arch may get higher. These changes can cause some parts of your feet to bear more weight. Those areas are then more likely to get corns and calluses.

CALLUSES

Calluses are hard areas of thick skin. If you don't have them trimmed, calluses can get very thick, break down, and turn into ulcers.

ULCERS

Ulcers are open sores or holes in the skin. Foot ulcers form most often over the ball of the foot or on the bottom of the big toe. They can also form on the sole, the heel, or the other toes.

Ulcers can be caused by a cut, callus, or blister that is not taken care of. Ulcers on the sides of a foot are usually caused by shoes that don't fit well.

An ulcer can be very painful. But if you have nerve damage, you may not feel it. If you ignore an ulcer, it may become infected. An infected ulcer can lead to gangrene and amputation.

GANGRENE AND AMPUTATION

Gangrene is death of tissues. Dead tissues turn black. There are two types of gangrene: dry and wet. Dry gangrene can be caused by poor circulation. Wet gangrene can be caused by an infected ulcer or infected dry gangrene.

Amputation is removal of the dead parts. It might mean you lose a toe, several toes, a foot, or part of a foot.

TO PREVENT FOOT PROBLEMS

- Keep blood glucose levels in your ideal range. High blood glucose levels make you more likely to get foot problems.
- If you smoke, try to quit. Smoking is hard on your blood vessels, limits blood flow to your feet, and causes wounds to heal more slowly. And if that isn't enough to make you want to quit, read this:

  Almost all people with diabetes who need amputations are smokers.

- Have your doctor check your feet for blood vessel, muscle, and nerve damage at least once a year.

- Check both your feet each day. Look all over your feet. If you cannot see well, have a friend or relative who can see well do it for you. Compare one foot to the other. Look for any of these foot problems:

Cuts	Blisters
Cracks	Breaks
Scratches	Calluses
Ingrown toenails	Swelling
Redness	Changes in color
Changes in shape	Pain
Cold spots	Loss of feeling
Hot spots	Corns
Ulcers	Dryness
Punctures	Peeling

- Call your doctor if you have a foot problem, no matter how minor. Take your shoes and socks off at every regular doctor visit to remind your doctor to check your feet.

- Keep your feet clean. Wash and dry them well. Don't forget to dry between your toes.

- Keep your feet out of water that is too hot or too cold. Test the water first with your elbow. And don't soak your feet. Soaking dries out your skin.

- Trim your toenails to follow the curve of your toe. If you can't trim them yourself, have a foot doctor do it.

- Put on clean socks each day. Pull your socks on gently. Or roll them on. Make sure your socks fit and there are no holes or bumpy areas in them. Buy socks without seams. Seams can rub your feet and cause blisters.

- Buy shoes that fit. Shoes that fit are comfortable when you buy them. Look for shoes with low heels and thick soles. Thick soles will cushion your feet and protect against injury. Pick shoes that are sturdy and give support. Make sure there is room for you to move your toes. Break in new shoes slowly.

- Check your shoes before you put them on. Make sure there are no stones, nails, paper clips, pins, or other sharp objects in them. Be sure the inside is smooth and free of tears or rough edges.

TIPS FOR COMMON FOOT PROBLEMS

If your feet are cold
> Wear warm socks. Do not use hot water bottles, heating pads, or electric blankets. They may burn your feet without you noticing.

If your feet are dry and scaly
> Use a moisturizer. But don't put the moisturizer between your toes. The extra moisture can lead to infection.

If your feet sweat a lot
> Try socks made of silk or thin polypropylene under your regular socks. They wick away sweat and help reduce friction. Be sure you have enough room in your shoes to fit both pairs of socks.

If you have calluses

Have them cut by your doctor or a foot doctor. Do not try to cut calluses yourself. Trying to cut calluses yourself can lead to ulcers and infections. Trying to remove calluses with over-the-counter chemicals can burn your skin.

If you have lost some of the feeling in your feet

Don't go barefoot. You could hurt your foot and not notice it. Your foot doctor may recommend shoe inserts or special shoes. If you are going swimming or wading, wear footwear made for water.

If your feet are tender

Try padded socks. They cushion and protect feet and help reduce callus buildup. They may make walking more comfortable. Be sure your shoe is large enough to fit this thicker sock. You may need extra-deep shoes.

If your feet are swollen

Try lace-up shoes. You can tighten or loosen them to fit the shape of your feet.

Gestational Diabetes

Gestational diabetes is high blood glucose levels that occur only in pregnant women who do not already have diabetes. It appears around the 24th week of pregnancy. At that time, the body is making large amounts of hormones to help the baby grow. It is thought that these hormones block insulin. When something in the body does not allow insulin to do its job, it is called insulin resistance.

In most pregnant women, the body makes enough insulin to overcome the insulin resistance. In some pregnant women, the insulin that is made cannot overcome the insulin resistance. These women have gestational diabetes. Most women with gestational diabetes have healthy babies. But close follow-up by a doctor is still important.

YOU ARE AT RISK FOR GESTATIONAL DIABETES IF

- You are overweight.
- You have a family history of diabetes.
- You have given birth to a baby weighing 9 pounds or more.

Gestational diabetes can be hard on you and your baby. If gestational diabetes is not treated, you and your baby are more likely to have the following problems.

MACROSOMIA

Macrosomia means large body. If your blood glucose is too high during pregnancy, the extra glucose in your blood goes into your baby. This causes your baby to make more insulin. The extra glucose and the extra insulin cause your baby to grow bigger and fatter than normal, making delivery harder. Babies who are larger than normal are more likely to have health problems.

HYPOGLYCEMIA

Hypoglycemia is low blood glucose. If your blood glucose is too high right before or during labor, your baby may have low blood glucose at birth. The extra glucose in your blood goes into your baby. This causes your baby to make more insulin.

After delivery, your baby no longer gets extra glucose from you. The extra insulin your baby made causes your baby's blood glucose level to fall. Hypoglycemia in your baby can be treated in the hospital right after birth.

JAUNDICE

Before your baby is born, he or she makes lots of red blood cells. After delivery, the baby no longer needs as many red blood cells. Your baby's liver breaks down the extra red blood cells and gets rid of them. If your baby's liver is not mature enough, it may have trouble doing this. The extra red blood cells and their breakdown products remain in the baby's body.

One breakdown product of red blood cells is bilirubin. Bilirubin colors your baby's skin yellow. This is called jaundice. Jaundice is simple to take care of in the hospital using special lights. But it can be dangerous if it is not treated. Ask your doctor about it before you take your baby home from the hospital.

HIGH KETONES

Ketones are made when your body burns stored fat for energy. Large amounts of ketones can harm you or your baby. Ketones are more likely to build up if you are not eating and drinking enough for both you and your baby. Be sure to eat all meals and snacks at your scheduled times.

PREECLAMPSIA

Preeclampsia (also called toxemia) is high blood pressure, swelling of your feet and lower legs, and leaking of protein into your urine during pregnancy. Other signs include headache, nausea, vomiting, abdominal pain, and blurred sight. If not treated, preeclampsia can cause seizures, coma, and death to you or your baby. Your doctor will watch for signs of preeclampsia.

URINARY TRACT INFECTION

When your blood glucose is high, you are more likely to get a urinary tract infection. Urinary tract infections are usually caused by bacteria. Bacteria grow much better and faster in high glucose.

Signs of a urinary tract infection include the need to urinate often, pain or burning when you urinate, cloudy or bloody urine, low back pain or abdominal pain, fever, and chills.

TO DETECT AND CARE FOR GESTATIONAL DIABETES

If you are pregnant, get tested for gestational diabetes between the 24th and 28th weeks of pregnancy. If you have gestational diabetes, your doctor may ask you to

- *Follow a meal plan.* A meal plan will help you avoid too high or too low blood glucose.
- *Follow an exercise program.* Exercise can help lower your blood glucose level.
- *Self-monitor your blood glucose.* This lets you know how your gestational diabetes-care plan is working.
- *Test your urine for ketones.* The earlier you detect ketones, the quicker you can stop them from getting worse. Ask your doctor when and how often you should test.

- *Take insulin.* When you have gestational diabetes, your body is not able to make and use all the insulin it needs for pregnancy. You may need to inject extra insulin. Diabetes pills are not used because they may harm the baby.

Gestational diabetes usually goes away after you give birth. But once you have had gestational diabetes, you are more likely to get type 1 or type 2 diabetes in the future.

Glycohemoglobin Test

Hemoglobin is a protein inside red blood cells. Hemoglobin carries oxygen from the lungs to all the cells of the body.

Like other proteins, hemoglobin can join with sugars, such as glucose. When this happens, it makes glycohemoglobin (GHb).

The more glucose there is in the blood, the more hemoglobin will join with it. Once joined, hemoglobin and glucose stay that way for the life of the red blood cell—about 4 months.

The GHb test measures the amount of glycohemoglobin in your red blood cells. The GHb test is done by a laboratory.

A sample of your blood is taken. The blood can be taken at any time of the day. It does not matter what food you last ate. It does not matter what your blood glucose level is at the time of the test.

WHAT THE GHb TEST CAN DO

- Tell you your average blood glucose level for the past 2 to 4 months. You can then see how your blood glucose control has been.
- Allow you to compare the GHb test results with blood glucose tests you have done yourself or tests your doctor has done. If the tests do not agree, you may need to change the way you test or when you test.

- Help you judge whether your diabetes-care plan is working. If your average blood glucose level is high, something in your plan may need to be changed.

- Show you how a change in your plan has affected your diabetes. Perhaps you started to exercise more. A GHb test can confirm the good effects exercise has had on your blood glucose control.

WHAT THE NUMBERS MEAN

There is more than one way to measure GHb. And there is more than one kind of GHb. One kind of GHb may be measured by several different tests. Because of this, GHb tests done at different laboratories may give different numbers.

If you change doctors or your doctor changes laboratories, be sure to find out what the numbers from the new laboratory mean. Usually, a higher GHb test number means you have a higher average blood glucose level. Work with your doctor or health care team to set GHb goals.

WHEN TO TEST

Have a GHb test when you find out you have diabetes. After that, do the following:

If you use insulin
Have the test done at least four times a year.

If you don't use insulin
Have the test done as your doctor recommends.

REASONS TO KEEP DOING SELF-TESTS

The GHb test can't replace the tests you do each day to measure the level of glucose in your blood (see Glucose, Self-Tests). Self-tests help you decide how to treat diabetes at that moment. What you do to keep daily blood glucose under control will show up in your GHb test results.

Health Care Team

A health care team is a group of health care professionals who help you manage your diabetes. The team includes you and may include a diabetes doctor (see Doctor), a nurse, a dietitian (see Dietitian), an exercise physiologist, a mental health professional, an eye doctor, a foot doctor, a dentist (see Dental Care), and a pharmacist. Your diabetes doctor may help you find the other members of the team.

Your team teaches you about diabetes and how to make diabetes care a part of your life. Your health care team depends on you to tell them how your diabetes-care plan is working and when you need their help. That is why you are the most important member of the team.

NURSE

Nurses teach and advise you on the day-to-day management of your diabetes. Nurses can teach you what diabetes is and how to

- Use diabetes pills.
- Use insulin.
- Give yourself insulin shots.
- Use an insulin pump.
- Test your blood glucose at home.
- Keep track of your diabetes control.

- Know the signs of low and high blood glucose.
- Take care of low or high blood glucose.
- Handle sick days.
- Stay healthy during pregnancy.

You may work with a diabetes nurse practitioner, a nurse clinician, or a nurse educator. Look for the initials RN after a nurse's name. RN stands for registered nurse (RN). Some nurses have a master's degree (MSN). Many nurses are certified diabetes educators (CDE).

CERTIFIED DIABETES EDUCATOR

The letters CDE after a person's name stand for certified diabetes educator. When you see these letters, you know the person is specially trained to teach or care for people with diabetes. These letters may come after the names of any of the people on your health care team.

A CDE is certified by the National Certification Board for Diabetes Educators and must stay up-to-date on diabetes care and treatment to remain certified. To find a diabetes educator in your area, call the Diabetes Educators Access Line at 1-800-832-6874.

MENTAL HEALTH PROFESSIONAL

Mental health professionals include social workers, psychologists, and psychiatrists. These people can help you with the emotional side of diabetes.

Look for a licensed clinical social worker (LCSW) with a master's degree in social work (MSW) and training in individual, group, and family therapy. Social workers can help you and your family cope with any stress or anxieties related to diabetes.

A clinical psychologist has a master's or doctoral degree in psychology and training in individual, group, and family psychotherapy. Clinical psychologists counsel patients with emotional problems.

A psychiatrist is a medical doctor who can provide counseling and prescribe drugs to treat physical causes for emotional problems.

EXERCISE PHYSIOLOGIST

An exercise physiologist is trained in the science of exercise and body conditioning. An exercise physiologist helps you plan a safe, effective exercise program.

Look for someone with a master's or doctoral degree in exercise physiology. Or find a licensed health care professional who has graduate training in exercise physiology. Certification from the American College of Sports Medicine is a good sign. Always get your diabetes doctor's approval on any exercise program.

EYE DOCTOR

Your eye doctor is either an ophthalmologist or an optometrist. Ophthalmologists are medical doctors who detect and treat eye diseases. They may prescribe eye medicines and perform eye surgery. Optometrists are not medical doctors. They are trained to examine the eye for vision problems and other minor problems. When you go to your eye doctor, find out

- Whether your eye doctor knows how to spot eye diseases and which ones
- How many of your eye doctor's patients have diabetes
- Whether your eye doctor performs eye surgery
- Whether your eye doctor will send regular reports to your diabetes doctor

FOOT DOCTOR

A foot doctor is called a podiatrist. A podiatrist is trained to treat foot and lower-leg problems. Podiatrists have a doctor of podiatric medicine (DPM) degree from a college of podiatry. They have also done a residency (hospital training) in podiatry. When you go to a foot doctor, find out

- How many of the foot doctor's patients have diabetes

- Whether the foot doctor knows the foot problems diabetes can cause
- Whether the foot doctor will work with your diabetes doctor

PHARMACIST

A pharmacist is trained in the chemistry of drugs and how drugs affect the body. A pharmacist has at least a bachelor of science degree in pharmacy or a doctor of pharmacy degree (PharmD).

Your pharmacist can help you in several ways. Most pharmacists offer free counseling. They can tell you

- How often to take your prescription drugs
- Whether to take your drugs with meals or on an empty stomach
- What side effects to watch for
- Whether to stay out of the sun
- What foods to avoid
- What other drugs might react with your new drug
- When to take a missed dose
- How to store your drugs
- What nonprescription drugs work best with your other drugs

OTHER TEAM MEMBERS

As your health changes, you may need other members on your team. If you plan to have a baby, you will need an obstetrician. If you have blood flow problems in your legs or feet, you may need a vascular surgeon. Your diabetes doctor can help you find the specialist you need.

Heart Attack

A heart attack occurs when blood flow to the heart is blocked. Without blood, the heart can't get the oxygen it needs. Part of the heart gets damaged or dies.

Blood flow can be cut off by a buildup of fat and cholesterol in the blood vessels that lead to the heart (see Blood Vessel Disease). Or blood flow can be cut off by a clot stuck in one of the blood vessels.

People with diabetes are more likely to have a heart attack than people without diabetes. High blood glucose may damage large blood vessels. You can't change the fact that you have diabetes. But there are things you can do to keep your heart healthy.

TO REDUCE YOUR RISK OF HEART ATTACK

- Control your diabetes. Keeping your blood glucose levels in your ideal range (see Blood Glucose) and meeting your GHb goals (see Glycohemoglobin Test) may prevent or delay blood vessel damage.

- Toss the cigarettes. Smoking narrows blood vessels and promotes the buildup of fat and cholesterol on blood vessel walls. Smoking makes blood clot faster.

- If you have high blood pressure, work with your doctor to control it. High blood pressure makes your heart work harder. This weakens your heart. You can bring your blood pressure down by eating healthfully, exercising, losing weight, and taking blood pressure drugs.

- Get a good low-fat, low-cholesterol cookbook and learn healthy, tasty ways to cook. High cholesterol can damage your blood vessels.
- Exercise for as little as 15 minutes a day three times a week! Try walking, biking, or swimming. These are aerobic exercises. Aerobic exercises use your heart, lungs, and large muscles.

     Aerobic exercises can lower blood pressure, lower LDL cholesterol and triglycerides, and raise HDL cholesterol. Aerobic exercises can improve overall heart health, promote weight loss, and reduce stress.

- If you are overweight, lose a few pounds! Losing even a little weight with diet and exercise lowers blood pressure and improves cholesterol levels.
- Remain calm in the face of stress (see Stress). Excess stress can raise blood pressure and blood glucose levels.
- Women should consider estrogen. If you have gone through menopause, ask your doctor about the female hormone estrogen. Estrogen may protect against heart disease. Estrogen can raise HDL cholesterol and may guard against blood clotting. Be aware that estrogen may increase the risk of breast or uterine cancer in some women.
- Be alert to the warning signs of a heart attack. Know what to do if the warning signs occur.

Warning signs of a heart attack

- Pain, tightness, pressure, or squeezing in the chest
- Pain that spreads to the neck, shoulders, arms, or jaw
- Shortness of breath, dizziness, or fainting
- Sweating, nausea

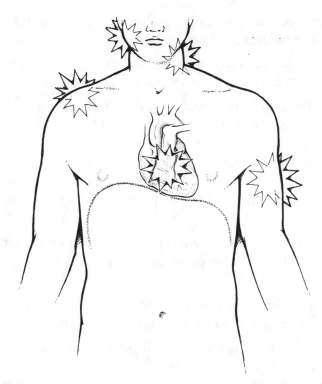

A heart attack may cause pain in the chest, neck, shoulders, arms, or jaw.

Special note: People with diabetes may have little or no pain. Be alert to shortness of breath or hiccups. The main sign may be high ketones (see Ketone Test).

IF YOU THINK YOU ARE HAVING A HEART ATTACK

1. Call 911 for an ambulance. Or have someone drive you to the nearest hospital with 24-hour emergency care for heart problems.

2. Tell those around you that you think you are having a heart attack. Otherwise, if you pass out, they may waste time trying to figure out what's wrong.

High Blood Pressure

Blood pressure is the force of your blood as it travels through your blood vessels. The higher your blood pressure, the more force on your blood vessels. Added force on your blood vessels can weaken and damage them.

Blood vessels nourish your organs and nerves. When blood vessels are weakened and damaged by high blood pressure, they don't nourish your organs and nerves as well as they should. Your organs and nerves become damaged.

People with diabetes are more likely to have high blood pressure than people without diabetes. High blood pressure increases your chances of having a heart attack or stroke (see Heart Attack, Stroke) and may worsen nephropathy (kidney disease) and retinopathy (an eye disease).

SIGNS OF HIGH BLOOD PRESSURE

High blood pressure usually has no signs. The only way to know if you have it is to get it checked. Your blood pressure is probably checked each time you visit your doctor.

Checking your blood pressure

Blood pressure can be checked with a device called a sphygmomanometer. A soft cuff is wrapped around your upper arm. The cuff is inflated until it tightens enough to stop the flow of blood. As the cuff is deflated, the force of the blood is heard through a stethoscope.

Blood pressure is reported as two numbers. The first number is the systolic pressure. Systolic pressure is the force of your blood when your heart contracts. The second number is the diastolic pressure. Diastolic pressure is the force of your blood when your heart relaxes.

A reading of 120 over 80 means a systolic pressure of 120 and a diastolic pressure of 80. It is written as 120/80 mm Hg. The mm Hg is the measurement—millimeters (mm) of mercury (Hg).

Hypertension is another name for high blood pressure. If you find out that your blood pressure is high, you and your doctor can take steps to control it. Your doctor will first try to find out the cause of your high blood pressure.

	Blood Pressure Reading (in mm Hg)
Normal blood pressure	Less than 130/85
High-normal blood pressure	130/85 to 139/89
Mild hypertension	140/90 to 159/99
Moderate hypertension	160/100 to 179/109
Severe hypertension	180/110 to 209/119
Very severe hypertension	More than 210/120

CAUSES OF HIGH BLOOD PRESSURE

Sometimes, there is a specific cause, such as a kidney problem, hormone disorder, pregnancy, or the use of birth control pills. When high blood pressure is linked to a specific cause, it is called secondary hypertension. If you have secondary hypertension, your doctor will treat the cause first.

Most of the time, there is no obvious cause for high blood pressure. When there is no obvious cause, it is called essential hypertension. If you have essential hypertension, there are things you can do to bring your blood pressure down without having to take drugs.

TO LOWER YOUR BLOOD PRESSURE

Lose excess weight. Losing even a little extra weight may be enough to return your blood pressure to normal. The only way to lose weight and to keep it off is to follow a weight-loss diet and an exercise program. Your doctor and dietitian can help you make a plan that you can live with.

Stop smoking. Smoking causes high blood pressure by damaging blood vessels. Stopping smoking can do more to lower your risk of hypertension-related death than taking blood pressure drugs.

Drink less alcohol. Drinking more than 2 ounces of alcohol a day may cause high blood pressure. Your doctor may advise you to drink no more than 1 ounce of alcohol a day. There is about 1 ounce of alcohol in one mixed drink, one glass of wine, or a can of beer.

Eat less salt. Avoiding your salt shaker and foods with added salt may be enough to lower your blood pressure. If your doctor wants you to try a low-sodium diet, plan one with a registered dietitian.

Reduce stress. Stress may aggravate high blood pressure by causing your blood vessels to constrict and your heart to work harder. For tips on reducing stress, see Stress.

If you are not able to bring your blood pressure down with these changes, your doctor will probably put you on drugs to lower your blood pressure.

Blood pressure drugs used most often in people with diabetes are ACE (angiotensin-converting enzyme) inhibitors, alpha-1-receptor blockers, calcium antagonists, and thiazide diuretics in small doses.

These blood pressure drugs do not raise blood glucose levels, but they all have side effects. Ask your doctor or pharmacist about them.

Impaired Glucose Tolerance

A person with impaired glucose tolerance has a blood glucose level that is higher than normal but lower than the level of someone with diabetes. Impaired glucose tolerance is not a type of diabetes. But if you have impaired glucose tolerance, you are more likely to get type 2 diabetes. Doctors used to call impaired glucose tolerance by many other names. You may hear these names:

A touch of sugar

Borderline diabetes

Chemical diabetes

Latent diabetes

Potential diabetes

Prediabetes

Subclinical diabetes

The correct name is impaired glucose tolerance. The only way to know for sure that you have impaired glucose tolerance is through the following blood tests that are done by your doctor.

FASTING BLOOD GLUCOSE TEST

In the fasting blood glucose test, your blood glucose level is measured when you have not eaten for 8 to 12 hours. That is why it is usually done first thing in the morning.

People without diabetes usually have a fasting blood glucose level lower than 110 mg/dl. People with fasting blood glucose levels higher than 126 mg/dl on two tests have diabetes.

People with a fasting blood glucose level less than 126 mg/dl but more than 110 mg/dl have impaired glucose tolerance.

ORAL GLUCOSE TOLERANCE TEST

In the oral glucose tolerance test, your blood glucose levels are measured five times in 3 hours. First, your blood glucose is measured when you have not eaten for 8 to 12 hours (same as the fasting blood glucose test).

Then you drink a liquid with 75 grams of glucose in it (100 grams for pregnant women). Your blood glucose is then measured after 30 minutes, 1 hour, 2 hours, and 3 hours.

In a person without diabetes, the blood glucose levels rise and then fall quickly. They are under 200 mg/dl every time they are measured.

In a person with diabetes, the glucose levels rise higher than normal and stay up longer. The blood glucose levels are over 200 mg/dl after 2 hours and at one of the other times.

In a person with impaired glucose tolerance, the blood glucose levels are between 140 and 200 mg/dl at 2 hours after the glucose drink and are higher than 200 mg/dl at one of the other times.

POSTPRANDIAL BLOOD GLUCOSE TEST

In the postprandial blood glucose test, your blood glucose level is measured at a certain time (usually 2 hours) after eating a meal.

People without diabetes have postprandial blood glucose levels less than 200 mg/dl. People with postprandial blood glucose levels greater than 200 mg/dl have diabetes.

People with postprandial blood glucose levels between 140 and 200 mg/dl may have impaired glucose tolerance.

YOU HAVE IMPAIRED GLUCOSE TOLERANCE IF

- Your fasting blood glucose test is less than 126 mg/dl but more than 110 mg/dl.

- Your oral glucose tolerance test is between 140 and 200 mg/dl at 2 hours after the glucose drink.

- At least one of your other oral glucose tolerance tests is higher than 200 mg/dl.

- Your postprandial blood glucose test is between 140 and 200 mg/dl.

Impaired glucose tolerance needs to be treated, even though you may never get diabetes. To be on the safe side, go back to your doctor at least once a year to have your blood glucose tested.

In the meantime, there are a few things you can do to help you return your blood glucose levels to normal:

- Lose weight (if you are overweight)

- Eat healthfully

- Exercise

Insulin

nsulin is a hormone that helps glucose get inside your body's cells. Your cells use glucose for energy. Insulin is made in the pancreas. Your pancreas lies behind your stomach.

If you have type 1 diabetes, your pancreas no longer makes insulin, or it makes only a tiny amount. That's why you need to take insulin.

If you have type 2 diabetes, your pancreas still makes insulin. But it doesn't make enough, or your body has a hard time using the insulin, or both. You may need to take diabetes pills or you may need to take insulin.

INSULIN SOURCES

There are two different sources of insulin: animals and bacteria. Animal (pork or pork/beef) insulin comes from the pancreases of dead pigs and cows. Human insulin is made with bacteria in a laboratory. It does not come from humans.

Today, in the United States, more people use human insulin than animal insulin. Animal insulin is more likely to cause allergies than human insulin. But many people do use animal insulin without problems.

INSULIN TYPES

There are several types of insulin. They are grouped by the way they act. Insulin's action has three parts: onset, peak time, and duration. Onset is how long insulin takes to start working. Peak time is when insulin is working its hardest. Duration is how long insulin keeps working. The times for onset, peak, and duration are given as ranges in the table below. There are two reasons for these ranges: 1) insulin may work slower or faster in you than in someone else, and 2) human insulin works faster than animal insulin.

	Fast-acting insulin	Short-acting insulin	Intermediate-acting insulin	Long-acting insulin
Onset	20 to 40 minutes	30 to 120 minutes	2 to 6 hours	6 to 14 hours
Peak	30 to 120 minutes	2 to 4 hours	4 to 14 hours	Minimal
Duration	4 to 6 hours	3 to 8 hours	10 to 24 hours	18 to 36 hours
Types	Lispro	Regular	NPH and Lente	Ultralente

INSULIN STRENGTH

Insulins come dissolved in liquids. The mixtures come in different strengths. Most people use U-100 insulin. This means that there are 100 units of insulin per milliliter of fluid. If you inject insulin, it is important to use a syringe that matches the strength of your insulin. For instance, if you use U-100 insulin, use a U-100 syringe.

INSULIN STORAGE

Insulin makers advise storing your insulin in the refrigerator. Do not put your insulin in the freezer or allow it to warm in the sun. Extreme temperatures can destroy insulin. Doctors say the bottle of insulin you are using can be left at room temperature for up to 1 month.

INSULIN SAFETY

Check the expiration date before opening your insulin. If the date has passed, don't use the insulin. If the date is yet to come, look closely at the insulin in the bottle. If you are looking at Regular insulin, it should be clear, with no floating pieces or color. If you are looking at NPH, Lente, or Ultralente insulin, it should be cloudy. But it should not have floating pieces or crystals.

If the insulin does not look as it should, return the unopened bottle of insulin to the place you bought it for an exchange or refund.

INSULIN THERAPY

Your doctor will help you plan what kinds of insulin to take, how much, and when. It is important to follow this plan closely. Your plan may be a standard or intensive one.

Standard insulin therapy means you take one or two insulin shots of the same dose at the same times each day. Often, you take one shot in the morning and one in the evening.

Standard therapy may work well for you, or it may leave your blood glucose levels too high. But you usually won't have severe high or low blood glucose levels.

Intensive insulin therapy means you take three or more insulin shots a day or use an insulin pump. You change your insulin dose to fit the results of your blood glucose tests, how much you are planning to eat, or what exercises you are going to do.

Intensive therapy aims to keep your blood glucose levels very close to normal. Because you are keeping your blood glucose levels lower, your chances of having severe low blood glucose are greater. You may also gain some weight.

Talk with your health care team about which insulin therapy is best for you. The best therapy is the one that helps you meet your blood glucose and glycohemoglobin test goals.

Insulin Pumps

An insulin pump is a battery-powered, computerized device about the size of a deck of cards. Inside the pump is a syringe of short-acting insulin with a gear-driven plunger. A thin tube, 21 to 43 inches long, is attached to the pump. At the other end of the tube is a needle or catheter. You insert the needle or catheter under your skin, usually in your abdomen or thigh. Insulin is delivered through the tube and needle or catheter into your body.

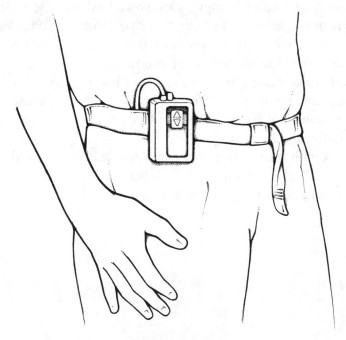

Insulin Pump

You program the pump. You tell it how much insulin you want and when you want it. You tell the pump to give you tiny amounts of short-acting insulin continuously throughout the day and night, just the way a normal pancreas would. Then you tell the pump to give you extra insulin just before you eat.

You wear an insulin pump pretty much all the time, either inside or outside your clothes. A pump may be waterproof or come with a waterproof case for showers and swimming.

You can, of course, take the pump off. If you'll have the pump off for more than 1 hour, you may need a shot of short-acting insulin. Check your blood glucose to be sure. Yes, you still need to test your blood glucose. At least four tests a day are recommended.

WHAT THE PUMP CAN DO FOR YOU

Get your blood glucose levels closer to normal. This is called tight control. If your insulin shots have not controlled your blood glucose levels, an insulin pump might work better for you.

Smooth out blood glucose swings. If you have frequent blood glucose swings, the insulin pump can help smooth them out.

Take care of the nighttime lows and the morning highs. Your body needs less insulin at night than at dawn. If you try to lower the dose of your evening insulin shot to avoid low blood glucose at night, you won't have enough insulin in the morning. Then you'll have high blood glucose when you wake up.

With an insulin pump, you can program it to give you less insulin at night and more insulin before dawn. That way you avoid nighttime low blood glucose and morning high blood glucose.

BE AWARE

Ketoacidosis. When your body has too little or no insulin, you risk getting ketoacidosis. Ketoacidosis is a dangerous buildup of ketones in your blood.

If the tube to your insulin pump gets blocked or twisted or the needle comes out, you won't be getting insulin, and you may not know it.

(Pumps do have alarms that signal when the tube is blocked, the insulin is low, or the battery is low. But they don't signal when the needle has come out.)

Ketones can start to build up in 1 hour. Ketoacidosis can develop in as little as 6 hours. Your best protection is to check your blood glucose levels often. If your blood glucose level is over 250 mg/dl, check your urine for ketones.

Infection. The place where the needle or catheter enters your body may become infected. To lessen your chances of infection, clean the area before you insert the needle or catheter, change sites within the area every 48 hours (see Insulin Shots), and use an antibiotic ointment and protective cover.

Skin allergy. You may have an allergic reaction around the needle or catheter site. Try nonallergenic tape or Teflon catheters.

COSTS AND INSURANCE

Pumps cost between $3,000 and $5,000. Supplies for a month, including blood glucose monitoring strips, cost about $300.

Medicare and some insurance companies will not pay either the cost of the pump or the cost for maintaining the pump. Insurance companies are more likely to pay the costs if your doctor explains your need for the pump to the insurance company.

If you think you may want a pump, talk to your doctor. Learning how to use a pump can take some time. Your doctor may want you to be in the hospital for a few days when you first get a pump so that you can learn all about how to use it.

Insulin Shots

nsulin cannot be taken in a pill. It would be broken down like food before it could work. Insulin needs to be injected under the skin, in the fat, to work well. Injecting into fat is much less painful than injecting into muscle. Besides, if you inject into muscle, the insulin will not work as well. Usually it will work too fast.

WHERE TO GIVE YOURSELF A SHOT

Areas. Areas are the places on your body where you can inject insulin. There are four good areas for insulin shots:

1. Your abdomen (anywhere except within 2 inches of the navel)

2. Your upper arms (outside part)

3. Your buttocks (anywhere)

4. Your thighs (front and outside parts, not inner thigh, not just above your knee)

These areas absorb insulin at different speeds. Your abdomen absorbs insulin the fastest. Your upper arms absorb insulin more slowly. Your buttocks and thighs absorb insulin even more slowly.

Depending on where you inject your insulin, it may act faster or slower. This can affect your blood glucose control.

You may prefer to take your shot in the same area so that you know how it will act. Some doctors suggest that you take all your shots in the abdomen. Others suggest that you choose your area according to how fast or slow you want the insulin to start working.

One plan is to inject your breakfast and lunch insulin doses into your arms and abdomen (the areas that absorb faster) and to inject your supper and bedtime doses into your buttocks and thighs (the areas that absorb slower). Your doctor may suggest another plan for you. Whatever plan you try, keep track of how your body responds by testing your blood glucose and recording the results.

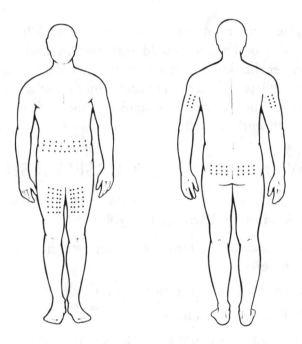

Sites for insulin shots

Sites. Pretend that each area is covered with circles that are 1 inch apart. Each circle is one site. The number of sites you have depends on how big your body is. The bigger your body, the more sites you have in each area.

Within each area, it is best to change sites with each shot. This is called site rotation. To rotate sites, you use a different circle for each shot until all the circles have been used up. Then you start all over again. If you take all your shots in the same place, you can damage the tissue under your skin.

HOW TO GIVE YOURSELF A SHOT

1. Wash your hands with soap and water. Dry them.

2. Clean the site with 70% isopropyl alcohol.

3. Wipe the top of the insulin vial with 70% isopropyl alcohol.

4. Gently roll the vial in your hands to mix the insulin. (You do not need to do this to short-acting insulin.)

5. Draw air into the syringe. Stop at the mark for the insulin dose you want. Inject the air into the vial. This prevents a vacuum.

6. Turn the bottle upside down. Draw insulin into the syringe. Stop at the mark for the number of units you want. When mixing types of insulin, draw the short-acting insulin first.

7. Check for air bubbles. If there are air bubbles, flick your forefinger against the upright syringe a couple of times to get them out.

8. Grasp a fold of skin.

9. Inject at a 90-degree angle. If you are thin, you may need to inject at a 45-degree angle to avoid muscle.

10. After you've removed the needle, apply pressure to the site for 5 to 8 seconds without rubbing.

Syringes for injecting insulin have tiny needles with a slick coating so that they go in easily. Most people find that insulin shots don't hurt too much, if done correctly.

TO MAKE THE SHOT
EVEN MORE COMFORTABLE

• Inject insulin at room temperature. Using cold insulin right from the refrigerator may make a shot hurt more.

• Make sure there are no air bubbles in the syringe before you inject the insulin.

• Wait until the alcohol you put on your skin is dry.

• Relax your muscles in the area.

• Puncture the skin quickly.

- Keep the needle in the same direction when you put it in and take it out.
- Use sharp, not dull, needles.

REUSING SYRINGES

Makers of disposable syringes recommend that they be used only once. The makers cannot guarantee that the syringe will stay sterile.

If you want to reuse syringes, check with your doctor first, then follow these tips. Recap the needle after each use to keep it clean. Don't try to clean it with alcohol. Alcohol may rub off the slick coating. Watch out for infection at the site.

Throw away the syringe when the needle is dull, has been bent, or has come into contact with any surface other than your skin.

DISPOSING OF SYRINGES

The best way to dispose of your syringes is to place them in a puncture-proof container with a lid that can be sealed shut before it is placed in the garbage.

Another way to dispose of needles is with a needle-clipping device that clips, catches, and keeps the needles in a closed compartment.

Some states require you to destroy used insulin syringes and needles. But be careful if you recap, bend, or break a needle—you or someone else could get pricked with it.

There may be special rules for getting rid of syringes and needles where you live. Ask your local garbage company or city or county waste authority what method meets their rules.

Insurance

Taking care of your diabetes can be costly. Health insurance plans vary on what parts of your diabetes care they will help pay for. Before you sign up for a health insurance plan, find out

- Whether visits to your diabetes doctor are covered
- How much the insurance pays for each doctor bill
- How much the insurance pays for a hospital stay
- Whether there is a limit on what you pay each year
- Whether there is a limit on what the insurance company pays each year
- Whether you will be covered right away or whether you will have to wait because you have diabetes (a preexisting condition)
- Whether the insurance will cover blood glucose meters, lancets, strips, insulin, syringes, insulin pumps, and other diabetes supplies
- Whether the insurance will help pay for diabetes educators or dietitians, mental health professionals, specialists, prescription drugs, and home care

If you work, your employer may offer you a group health plan. Group plans are usually open to all employees. Your employer may pay most or all of the cost (premium) for you. For an additional fee, these plans may also cover your spouse and children. Group plans may be of two types: fee-for-service plans or prepaid managed-care plans.

FEE-FOR-SERVICE PLANS

In a fee-for-service plan, you or your employer pays a yearly fee to an insurance company. The insurance company then pays for all or part of the cost of your medical care. Usually, the insurance company will start paying after you have paid a small amount of the cost, called a deductible. The biggest advantage of a fee-for-service plan is that you pick the health care providers you want to go to.

MANAGED-CARE PLANS

Managed care is a general term for an organized group of health care providers. Managed-care plans include health maintenance organizations (HMOs), preferred provider organizations (PPOs), and exclusive provider organizations (EPOs). The biggest advantage of managed-care plans is that costs are usually lower for you.

Health maintenance organizations (HMOs)

An HMO is an organization that hires or contracts with health care professionals to provide a wide range of medical services to individuals and families. Most of the cost of your medical care is covered by a fee paid by you and/or your employer.

Depending on the type of HMO, you may or may not have to satisfy a deductible and/or pay a co-payment at each visit. Also depending on the type of HMO, you may or may not be covered if you go to a provider who is outside the HMO. Before you sign up, be sure to find out how the HMO works.

Preferred provider organizations (PPOs)

A PPO is a list of health care providers. The list is prepared and provided by an insurance company. The providers on the list are "preferred" because they have agreed with an insurer to discount their fees.

The preferred providers are paid by the insurer and by a small co-payment from you when you go to them. You may have to pay a small deductible. You may choose to go to a provider who does not belong to the PPO, but then you pay more.

Exclusive provider organizations (EPOs)

An EPO is like a PPO with an important difference. If you choose to go to a provider who does not belong to the EPO, you pay the total bill.

COBRA

COBRA stands for Consolidated Omnibus Budget Reconciliation Act. This federal law lets some people keep health insurance coverage for a limited time when they would otherwise lose it. You may need health insurance coverage when you are between jobs, when you go from full-time to part-time status, or when you retire. You may want health insurance coverage while you wait for a preexisting condition clause to expire at a new job. Your dependents may need health insurance coverage if you die or if you and your spouse separate or divorce.

If you want to stay covered, you must notify your employer in writing within 60 days after the event that will cause you to lose coverage. You pay the share of the premium you paid before. You usually must pay your employer's share, too. You often pay a small service fee as well.

Coverage begins the day you would have lost health insurance. Coverage may last for up to 18 months after you leave your job. If you are disabled, coverage may last up to 29 months. Your dependents may keep coverage for up to 36 months.

When your coverage is over, your employer may allow you to convert to an individual policy. Individual coverage is costly, but this option keeps you insured.

Private companies and state and local government offices are covered by COBRA. Employers with fewer than 20 employees, the federal government, and churches are not covered by COBRA. For more information on COBRA, call the COBRA Hot Line at 202-219-8776.

THE HEALTH INSURANCE PORTABILITY AND ACCOUNTABILITY ACT OF 1996

The Health Insurance Portability and Accountability Act of 1996 (effective 1 July 1997) makes it easier for people with diabetes to get and keep their health insurance.

According to the Act, insurers and employers may not make insurance rules that discriminate against workers because of their health.

And all workers eligible for a particular health insurance plan must be offered enrollment at the same price.

Insurers who sell individual policies must offer an individual policy without preexisting condition exclusions to anyone who 1) has had continuous coverage in a group plan for the previous 18 months, 2) is not currently eligible for coverage under any group plan, and 3) has used up COBRA coverage (see above).

Another part of the Act helps you keep coverage when you change jobs. If you have had diabetes for more than 6 months and have had continuous coverage in an insurance plan, and then leave your job, you cannot be denied coverage by your new employer because of a preexisting condition. If, however, you have been recently diagnosed, that is, up to 6 months ago, and you change jobs, your new employer may refuse or limit your health insurance coverage for 12 months. This is a one-time only waiting period, and it can be reduced by the number of months you had continuos coverage at your previous job. For example, say you were diagnosed with diabetes while employed and covered by your employer's health insurance plan. Five months after the diagnosis, you change jobs. Your new employer may limit or deny your health insurance coverage for the remainder of the 12-month waiting period, or 7 months.

MEDICARE

Medicare is a federal health insurance program for people aged 65 years and older and for people who cannot work because of certain disabilities. There are two parts to Medicare: Part A and Part B.

Part A helps to pay bills for medical care provided in hospitals, skilled nursing facilities, hospices (for people who are dying), and homes.

Part B helps to pay for doctor visits, ambulance services, lab tests, outpatient hospital services, outpatient physical therapy and speech pathology services, and medical equipment and supplies.

Most people covered by Medicare get Part A. You can get Part B by paying a monthly fee. Both parts have deductibles and co-payments that you pay. For more information on Medicare, call the Medicare Hot Line at 1-800-638-6833.

MEDIGAP

Medigap plans cover some of what Medicare doesn't, such as prescription drugs, Medicare deductibles, foreign travel emergencies, preventive care, or other costs.

The federal government has defined 10 standard Medigap plans. Some plans may not be offered in your state. Medigap plans are sold by private insurance companies. Prices for the same plan vary with insurance companies. Check prices with several insurance companies before you buy a Medigap plan.

MEDICAID

If your income is very low, you might be able to get Medicaid. Medicaid is a federal and state assistance program. Each state decides what income level it thinks is very low. And each state decides what medical services and supplies to cover. Call your state's Medicaid office to find out if you qualify and what health costs are covered.

SOCIAL SECURITY DISABILITY INSURANCE

If you lose your job because you are disabled, you may be able to get Social Security Disability Insurance. This insurance covers people under age 65 who have worked for pay recently and who are now disabled.

Social Security has a list of disabilities. If you have a disability on that list and earn less than $500 a month, you are considered disabled. For more information, call Social Security on weekdays at 1-800-772-1213.

Ketone Test

Ketones are waste products that are made when your body burns stored fat for energy. Your body burns fat when it can't get glucose to use for energy. This can happen in people with diabetes for several reasons.

HIGH GLUCOSE

High glucose means you have too much glucose and not enough insulin in your blood. Your body needs insulin to use glucose for energy. If you don't have enough insulin, your body starts to burn fat for energy.

LOW GLUCOSE

Low glucose means you have too much insulin and not enough glucose in your blood. Glucose comes from food you eat. Maybe you did not eat enough food. When your body is not getting enough glucose, it starts to burn fat for energy.

EXERCISE

When you exercise, your body needs lots of energy. If you don't have enough insulin or enough glucose when you exercise, your body will burn too much fat.

STRESS

It may be a physical stress, like surgery. Or it may be a mental stress, like an exam. Whatever kind of stress you're under, your body needs energy to handle it. Your body needs so much energy that it will burn fat if you don't have enough glucose.

ILLNESS

You may have a cold, a sore throat, a fever, or an infection. You may have diarrhea or an upset stomach. When you are sick, your body needs extra energy to fight it. Your body may get some of that extra energy from fat.

PREGNANCY

When you are pregnant, your body needs to provide energy for two. If you are not eating enough, your body may turn to fat for the energy it needs.

WHAT KETONES CAN DO TO YOUR BODY

If your body burns too much fat too quickly, high levels of ketones can build up in your blood. Ketones make your blood more acidic. Acidic blood upsets your body's chemical balance. Ketones are passed into your urine.

If blood glucose is high, glucose also passes into your urine. Glucose makes your urine thick. Your body pulls fluid from everywhere to thin out the urine. You make lots of urine. You can get dehydrated.

If you are dehydrated and your ketones are high, you may get ketoacidosis. This is life-threatening. Ketoacidosis can develop in as little as 6 hours.

Most people who get ketoacidosis have type 1 diabetes. But everyone with diabetes needs to be alert for the signs of it.

SIGNS OF KETOACIDOSIS

Dry mouth	Dry, flushed skin
Great thirst	Fever
Fruity breath	Fatigue
Loss of appetite	Drowsiness
Stomach pain	Frequent urination
Nausea	Labored breathing
Vomiting	

TEST FOR KETONES

If you have signs of ketoacidosis or are ill, pregnant, or under stress, test your urine for ketones. Test also if your blood glucose is over 240 mg/dl, especially if you are going to exercise.

Urine tests for ketones come in three forms: tapes, tablets, and test strips. Urine ketone test kits are available at your local pharmacy. You don't need a prescription. Follow the directions provided in the package. Go over the correct way to test with your doctor or nurse.

Most urine tests go like this:

1. Dip the test strip or tape in a sample of your urine, OR urinate on the test strip or tape, OR put drops of urine on the tablet.

2. Wait to see if the tape, strip, or tablet changes color. The directions will tell you how long to wait. You may need to wait anywhere from 10 seconds to 2 minutes.

3. Match the tape, strip, or tablet color to the color chart provided.

4. Record your results. You should record the type of test, the date and time, the result, and anything unusual. For example, maybe you forgot to take your insulin.

What to do with the results

If the result shows trace or small amounts of ketones

1. Drink a glass of water every hour.

2. Test blood glucose and ketones every 3 or 4 hours.

3. If blood glucose and ketone numbers are not going down after two tests, call your doctor.

If the result shows moderate or large amounts of ketones

1. Call your doctor right away! Don't wait. If you wait, your ketone levels may go higher.

HHNS

HHNS is an abbreviation for hyperosmolar hyperglycemic nonketotic syndrome. It is a life-threatening condition of high blood glucose and severe dehydration. Anyone with type 2 diabetes can develop HHNS. But HHNS doesn't just happen. It is usually brought on by something else, such as an illness, a heart attack, or extensive burns.

In HHNS, blood glucose levels rise, and your body tries to get rid of the excess glucose by passing it into your urine. This makes your urine thicker. Fluids are pulled from all over your body to thin out the urine. You make lots of urine, and you have to urinate more often. You also get very thirsty. If you don't drink enough fluids at this point, you can get dehydrated.

If HHNS continues, the severe dehydration will lead to seizures, coma, and eventually death. HHNS usually takes days or even several weeks to develop. When you are sick, drink a glassful of fluid (alcohol-free and caffeine-free) every hour, and test your blood glucose more often.

WARNING SIGNS

Blood glucose level over 600 mg/dl	High fever (105°F, for example)
Dry, parched mouth	Sleepiness or confusion
Extreme thirst (although this may gradually disappear)	Loss of vision
	Hallucinations
Warm, dry skin that does not sweat	Weakness on one side of your body

Kidney Disease

Kidneys clean your blood. Your blood flows through filters in your kidneys. In healthy kidneys, the filters let wastes pass out to your urine while keeping good and useful things in your blood. But diabetes can make your kidneys unhealthy. Unhealthy kidneys can get kidney disease.

Kidney disease is also called nephropathy. In nephropathy,

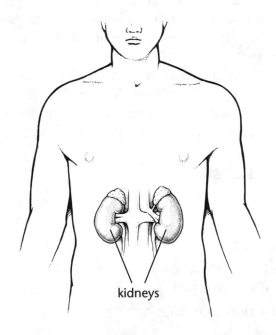

kidneys

Kidneys are located on either side of the small of your back.

kidneys go from being overworked, to leaky, to not being able to filter, and finally, to failure.

OVERWORKED FILTERS

People with diabetes often have high levels of glucose in their blood. High levels of glucose make your kidneys filter blood more often than is really needed. This extra work can be hard on the filters. The filters can become overworked.

LEAKY FILTERS

Overworked filters may start to leak. One thing they can leak is a protein called albumin. The filters leak albumin into the urine. A small amount of albumin in the urine is the first outward sign of kidney damage. As more and more albumin leaks into the urine, the level of albumin in the blood falls.

VERY LEAKY FILTERS

One job of albumin is to hold water in the blood. If there is not enough albumin in the blood, water leaks out of the blood vessels. The water can end up in the ankles, the abdomen, and the chest.

Water in your ankles makes them swell. Water in your abdomen causes bloating. Water in your chest makes it hard to breathe. These may be the first physical signs that something is wrong with your kidneys.

FILTERS THAT DON'T FILTER WELL

After a time, some of the overworked leaky filters just stop working. This makes more work for the filters that are still good. At first, the good filters work harder to make up for the ones that have stopped. Then they, too, stop working.

As more filters stop, fewer filters are left to do the work. Eventually, none of the filters are able to remove wastes. Wastes build up in the blood.

FILTERS THAT FAIL

Wastes in the blood rise to toxic levels when the kidneys' filters are no longer working. This is called kidney failure or end-stage renal disease.

SIGNS OF KIDNEY FAILURE

Foul taste in the mouth	Restless legs
Poor appetite	Loss of sleep at night
Upset stomach	Fatigue during the day
Throwing up	Lack of concentration
Easy bruising	

A person with kidney failure needs to have either a kidney transplant or dialysis. In a kidney transplant, the person gets a new kidney from someone else. In dialysis, a solution or a machine cleans the blood. There are steps you can take to slow down kidney disease before kidney failure.

TO SLOW DOWN KIDNEY DISEASE

- *Keep your blood glucose levels close to normal.* Keeping your blood glucose levels close to normal is known as tight control. Tight blood glucose control, more than anything else, can slow the progress of kidney disease.

- *Have your doctor check how your kidneys are working.* There are urine tests and blood tests to detect the start and progress of kidney disease. Two blood tests (blood urea nitrogen and serum creatinine) and one urine test (creatinine clearance) tell how well your kidneys are getting rid of wastes. Another urine test (albumin excretion rate) shows whether your kidneys are leaking.

- *Have your eyes checked for eye disease.* Most people with diabetes who get kidney disease also have eye problems. Damage to the eyes can be spotted earlier than damage to the kidneys.

- *Keep an eye on your blood pressure.* When your kidneys' filters are not working well, extra salt and water stay in the body. This can raise blood pressure. High blood pressure makes the kidneys work harder, and they can get more damaged.

If you have high blood pressure, try to get it under 130/85 mm Hg. Some ways to bring blood pressure down are by losing weight, eating less salt, and avoiding alcohol.

Ask your doctor about drugs to lower blood pressure. One class of blood pressure drugs, called ACE (angiotensin-converting enzyme) inhibitors, may even slow the progress of kidney disease.

- *Limit protein.* Most researchers have found that if you limit the amount of protein you eat, you may slow down kidney disease. But experts have not agreed on how much protein is best.

  Most Americans get about 14 to 18 percent of their daily calories from protein. The American Diabetes Association recommends that people with signs of kidney disease get about 10 percent of their daily calories from protein.

  Foods high in protein include meat, fish, poultry, eggs, milk, cheese, legumes, whole grains, and nuts and seeds. Work with a dietitian to make a low-protein meal plan.

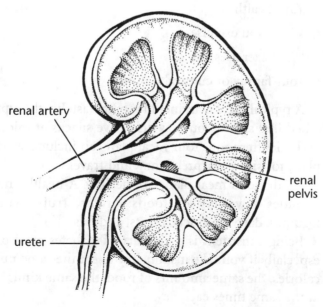

renal artery

renal pelvis

ureter

Detail of a kidney

Meal Planning

Most people with diabetes have a meal plan. A meal plan tells you what to eat, how much to eat, and when to eat. A dietitian helps you make your meal plan. Together, you work out a meal plan that is right for you. It will be based on

- What you like to eat and drink
- When you like to eat and drink
- How many calories you need
- Your daily schedule
- Your health
- When you exercise
- What exercises you do
- Your family or cultural customs

A typical meal plan includes breakfast, lunch, supper, and a bedtime snack. You may also have snacks at midmorning and midafternoon. Your meal plan can include special meal plans for sick days, pregnancy, and travel.

All diabetes meal plans are healthy. A healthy meal plan includes a variety of foods: grains, fruits, vegetables, legumes, dairy products, meats, and fats.

Being consistent is a big part of diabetes meal planning, especially if you take insulin. Try to eat the same number of calories, the same amounts of food, the same kinds of foods, at the same times each day.

Doing this helps you control your blood glucose levels. If you skip a meal or snack, you risk large swings in your blood glucose levels.

A meal plan can help you meet your other health goals as well. Your other health goals may include

- Better blood fat levels
- Normal blood pressure
- A healthy weight

Three meal-planning tools for people with diabetes are Exchange Lists, carbohydrate counting, and the Food Pyramid.

EXCHANGE LISTS

Exchange lists are lists of foods. Foods are listed together because they are alike. One serving of any of the foods on a list has about the same amount of carbohydrate, protein, fat, and calories. Any food on a list may be "exchanged" or traded for any other food on the same list.

EXCHANGE LISTS

Carbohydrate Group	Fat Group
1. Starch	10. Monounsaturated Fats
2. Fruit	11. Polyunsaturated Fats
3. Milk	12. Saturated Fats
4. Other Carbohydrates	
5. Vegetable	
Meat and Meat Substitutes	**Other Lists**
6. Very Lean	13. Free Foods
7. Lean	14. Combination Foods
8. Medium Fat	15. Fast Foods
9. High Fat	

Your dietitian can help you work out a plan using the exchange lists. The meal plan will tell you the number of food exchanges you can eat at each meal and snack. You then choose foods that add up to those exchanges.

With exchange lists, you do not need to count nutrients. As long as you follow your plan, you are eating a balanced diet. In *Exchange Lists for Meal Planning,* published by the American Diabetes Association and The American Dietetic Association, there are 3 main groups and 15 exchange lists.

The Other Carbohydrates list includes baked goods, frozen desserts, jams and jellies, syrups, and potato and tortilla chips. Although these foods contain added sugars or fat, you can learn how to substitute them for foods on the Starch, Fruit, or Milk lists. Keep in mind that foods on the Other Carbohydrates list are not as nutritious as those on the other lists.

Foods on the Free Foods list have less than 20 calories or less than 5 grams of carbohydrate per serving. They include fat-free or reduced-fat foods, sugar-free or low-sugar foods, no-calorie drinks (coffee, tea), and condiments (catsup, mustard) and seasonings (garlic, herbs). Free Foods are not likely to affect your blood glucose level if you follow the Exchange List guidelines for eating them.

CARBOHYDRATE COUNTING

When you eat a healthy meal or snack, it is usually a mixture of carbohydrate, protein, and fat. However, your body changes carbohydrate into glucose faster than it changes protein and fat into glucose.

In carbohydrate counting, you count foods that are mostly carbohydrate. These include starches (breads, cereals, pasta), fruits and fruit juices, milk, yogurt, ice cream, and sugars (honey, syrup). You do not count vegetables, meats, or fats. These foods have very little carbohydrate in them.

You can find out how much carbohydrate a food has by looking at the Exchange Lists, carbohydrate-counting books, and the Nutrition Facts on food labels (see Food Labeling) and by asking your dietitian.

Knowing how much carbohydrate a food has can help you control your blood glucose levels. If you have type 1 diabetes, and take Regular insulin, you can learn to adjust your insulin dose to cover the amount of carbohydrate you eat. If you have type 2 diabetes, you can learn to eat the same amount of carbohydrate each day.

FOOD PYRAMID

For years, the guide to healthy eating was the Basic Four Food Groups. But in 1992, the United States Department of Agriculture (USDA) changed the four food groups into six food groups. And they put the six food groups into sections of a pyramid. They called it the Food Guide Pyramid.

In 1995, The American Dietetic Association and the American Diabetes Association adapted the USDA Food Guide Pyramid into a pyramid just for people with diabetes. It is called the Diabetes Food Pyramid.

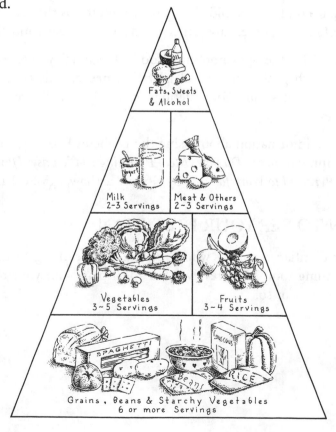

The pyramid tells you the daily number of servings to eat from the first five food groups. Your dietitian can help you learn how to divide these servings into the number of meals and snacks you eat in a day.

Using the Diabetes Food Pyramid

When using the pyramid, keep these three things in mind:

Variety. Eat a wide variety of foods from the food groups to get all the nutrients you need. For instance, eat more than one kind of vegetable.

Balance. Eat larger amounts and more servings from food groups that take up more space on the pyramid. The three food groups that take up more space are 1) grains, beans, and starchy vegetables; 2) vegetables; and 3) fruits.

Eat smaller amounts and fewer servings from food groups that take up less space on the pyramid. The three food groups that take up less space are 1) milk, 2) meat and others, and 3) fats, sweets, and alcohol.

Moderation. Eat the right amount of food. How much you eat depends on your health goals, calorie and nutrition needs, activity level, and insulin or diabetes pills. Your dietitian can help you figure out how much to eat.

For more information about using the Diabetes Food Pyramid as a meal-planning tool, see *Diabetes Meal Planning Made Easy: How to Put the Food Pyramid to Work for You,* by Hope Warshaw, MMSc, RD, CDE.

WHEN TO SEE YOUR DIETITIAN

See your dietitian regularly when you are first learning to use your meal-planning tool. Then review your meal plan with your dietitian every 6 months or so.

Nerve Damage

Nerve damage is called neuropathy. Neuropathy affects the nerves outside your brain and spinal cord. These are called peripheral nerves. There are three types of peripheral nerves: motor, sensory, and autonomic. Neuropathy can affect any of these nerves.

MOTOR NERVES

Motor nerves control your voluntary movement. Voluntary movements are those you make yourself do, like sitting, standing, and walking. Damage to the motor nerves can make your muscles weak and not able to do these things.

SENSORY NERVES

Sensory nerves allow you to feel and touch. Sensory nerves tell you if something is hot or cold. With sensory nerves, you can feel whether something is smooth or rough, soft or hard. Sensory nerves also let you feel pain. Damage to the sensory nerves can cause a loss of feeling.

AUTONOMIC NERVES

Autonomic nerves control involuntary activities. Involuntary activities are those your body does without you having to tell it to. You do not have to tell your lungs to breathe in and out or your heart to beat. You do not have to tell your stomach to digest food. Damage to the autonomic nerves can make it hard for your body's organs to work.

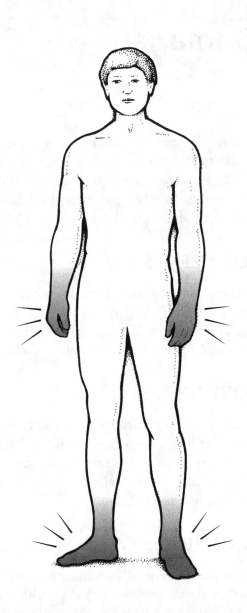

Distal symmetric polyneuropathy can
affect your feet, legs, or hands.

There are many types of neuropathy. Two of the most common are distal symmetric polyneuropathy and autonomic neuropathy.

DISTAL SYMMETRIC POLYNEUROPATHY

Distal symmetric polyneuropathy is nerve damage in the feet and legs and sometimes in the hands. Distal means it affects parts of the body that are far from the trunk. Symmetric means it occurs on both sides of the body. Polyneuropathy means that more than one nerve is damaged.

Signs of nerve damage to the feet, legs, or hands

- Coldness, numbness
- Tingling, burning
- Itching, prickling
- Sensation of bugs crawling over your skin
- Sensation of walking on a strange surface
- Deep aching
- Overly sensitive skin
- Pain on contact with sheets or clothing
- Electric shock–like sensations
- Jabs of needlelike pain

If you feel any of these signs, tell your doctor. The signs of nerve damage to the feet, legs, or hands tend to be worse at night. Signs often get better if you get out of bed and walk around a bit.

AUTONOMIC NEUROPATHY

Your autonomic nerves control your heart, lungs, blood vessels, stomach, intestines, bladder, and sex organs. Nerve damage to your heart can affect your heart rate and blood pressure. You may feel short of breath. Your heart may pound hard and fast when you are at rest. You may get dizzy or feel faint when you stand up quickly. Your ankles may swell. You may tire easily.

Nerve damage to your stomach affects digestion. This can cause you to feel bloated or full after eating even a small meal. You may feel sick to your stomach and vomit. When you vomit, you may see undigested food that you ate more than one meal before.

Damage to nerves in your intestines can cause diarrhea or constipation. If the nerves in your bladder are damaged, you will not be able to tell when your bladder is full of urine.

When you can't sense that your bladder is full, you don't go to the bathroom. Not going to the bathroom often enough can cause problems. You may dribble or wet yourself. Or the urine that stays in your bladder may cause a urinary tract infection.

Signs of a urinary tract infection include the need to urinate often, pain or burning when you urinate, cloudy or bloody urine, low back pain or abdominal pain, fever, and chills.

Nerve damage to sex organs can cause a loss of feeling or response during sex for both men and women (see Sex and Diabetes). *If you have any of these signs, see your doctor right away.*

TO PREVENT OR LESSEN NERVE DAMAGE

Keep blood glucose levels close to normal. When you have too much glucose in your blood, a lot of it goes into your nerve cells. Once inside nerve cells, this excess glucose forms sugar alcohols. The sugar alcohols build up, and your nerve cells don't work as well. After years of too much glucose, the nerves become damaged.

Stop smoking. Your nerves are fed by small blood vessels. Smoking damages these small blood vessels. Damaged blood vessels don't get oxygen to your nerves. Nerves without oxygen get damaged. If you already have nerve damage, smoking will make it worse.

Drink less alcohol. Drinking too much alcohol may cause nerve damage. If you already have nerve damage, drinking alcohol will make it worse.

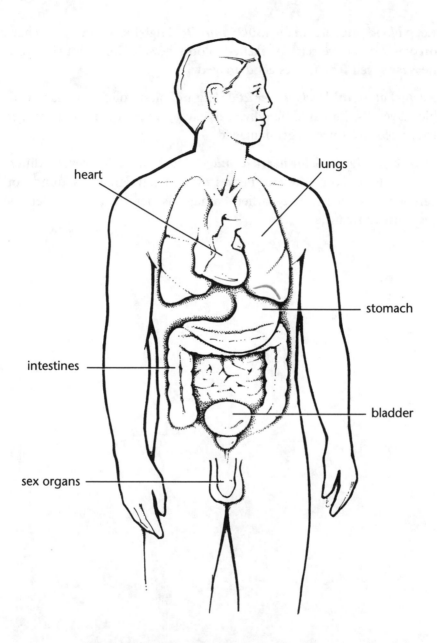

heart

lungs

stomach

intestines

bladder

sex organs

Autonomic neuropathy can affect your
heart, lungs, blood vessels, stomach, intestines,
bladder, or sex organs.

Keep blood pressure under 130/85 mm Hg. High blood pressure is hard on your blood vessels. Weakened blood vessels don't nourish your nerves as well. The nerves get damaged.

Keep cholesterol levels under 200. High cholesterol can damage your blood vessels. Damaged blood vessels can't give your nerves the oxygen they need. Your nerves get damaged.

Have a yearly check for nerve damage. A doctor can do several different tests to find out how your nerves are doing. If damage is found, you can get treatments. The earlier damage is detected, the better the response to treatment.

Nutrition

Nutrition means getting nutrients—protein, carbohydrates, fats, vitamins, and minerals—from what you eat and drink. What you eat and drink will affect your blood glucose level and your weight.

The American Diabetes Association (ADA) sets nutrition guidelines for people with diabetes. These guidelines help you make food choices. Many of these guidelines are the same for people without diabetes.

CALORIES

Calories are a measure of the energy you can get from food. Carbohydrates, protein, and fat are the main sources of calories in your diet.

One gram of carbohydrate has 4 calories. One gram of protein also has 4 calories. One gram of fat has 9 calories. Fat has more than twice as many calories as carbohydrate or protein.

Your food plan (see Meal Planning) will tell you how many calories you need to eat to stay at a healthy weight. This weight may not be your ideal weight but one that you can maintain.

CARBOHYDRATE

Carbohydrates provide your body with energy. Your body breaks down carbohydrates into glucose. ADA recommends that you and your health care team decide exactly how much carbohydrate you will eat in a day. Knowing this can help you better predict what your blood glucose is going to do.

You might get 50 percent or more of your daily calories from carbohydrates. Your dietitian will probably encourage you to eat more complex carbohydrates, like those in fruits, vegetables, and whole grains. Complex carbohydrates have more nutrients than simple carbohydrates, like honey and molasses.

CHOLESTEROL

Your liver makes cholesterol. And you get cholesterol from the animal foods you eat. ADA recommends that you eat less than 300 milligrams of cholesterol per day. If you have high LDL cholesterol levels, eat less than 200 milligrams per day.

FAT

There are two main kinds of fat in food: saturated and unsaturated. Saturated fats are found in animal foods and some plant foods. They are solid at room temperature. Unsaturated fats are found in plant foods. They are liquid at room temperature. Saturated fats raise your cholesterol level. Unsaturated fats lower your cholesterol level. Most people need to eat less saturated fat.

If your blood fat levels are normal and you are not overweight
    Get 30 percent or less of calories from fat.
    Get less than 10 percent of calories from saturated fat.

If you have high LDL cholesterol levels
    Get 30 percent or less of calories from fat.
    Get less than 7 percent of calories from saturated fat.

If you are overweight
    Get 20 to 25 percent of calories from fat.

FIBER

Fiber is the part of plants that your body can't digest. Fiber helps carry excess cholesterol out of your body and can protect your colon and intestines from diseases. ADA recommends that you get 20 to 35 grams of fiber per day. This recommendation is the same whether you have diabetes or not.

Try to get your fiber from a wide variety of foods. Fiber is found in fruits, vegetables, legumes (beans, peas, and lentils), and whole grains.

PROTEIN

Your body uses protein to make blood cells, body tissues, and hormones. ADA recommends that you get 10 to 20 percent of your daily calories from protein. If you have kidney disease, ADA recommends that you get about 10 percent of your daily calories from protein.

You can get your protein from both animal and plant foods. Foods that are high in protein include fish, poultry, meat, milk, legumes, whole grains, and nuts and seeds.

SODIUM

Sodium is salt. You may be more or less sensitive to sodium than someone else. One general rule is to get no more than 1 milligram of sodium for each calorie you eat in a day. For example, if you are on a 2,000-calorie diet, you would get no more than 2,000 milligrams of sodium each day. ADA recommends that

If you have normal blood pressure
   Get no more than 2,400 to 3,000 milligrams of sodium per day.

If you have mild to moderately high blood pressure
   Get 2,400 milligrams or less of sodium per day.

If you have high blood pressure and kidney disease
   Get 2,000 milligrams or less of sodium per day.

Oral Agents

Oral agents are pills that help you control your blood glucose levels. They are not insulin. Oral agents are for people with type 2 diabetes.

Doctors may prescribe oral agents for people who are not able to keep their blood glucose at safe levels with diet and exercise.

SULFONYLUREAS

You may be prescribed glyburide, tolbutamide, tolazamide, chlorpropamide, acetohexamide, glipizide, or glimepiride. These sulfonylureas help your body send out more of its own insulin. They also help your body respond to insulin. And they tell your liver to stop putting stored glucose into your blood. These actions lower your blood glucose. Sometimes sulfonylureas make your blood glucose go too low. They may also make it easier for you to gain weight.

Possible side effects of sulfonylureas

- Nausea
- Vomiting
- Rash
- Itching

METFORMIN

You may be prescribed metformin. Metformin belongs to a class of drugs called biguanides. Metformin causes your liver to release stored glucose more slowly. Metformin may also help your body respond to insulin. These actions keep your blood glucose levels more even. Metformin does not help your body send out more insulin. Because of this, there is less chance of low blood glucose and weight gain.

Possible side effects of metformin

- Metallic taste in your mouth
- Upset stomach
- Nausea
- Loss of appetite
- Diarrhea

These side effects usually go away after a short time. Metformin can cause lactic acidosis in people with heart, kidney, or liver disease. Lactic acidosis is a life-threatening buildup of acid in the blood. If you have heart, kidney, or liver disease, do not take metformin.

ACARBOSE

You may be prescribed acarbose. Acarbose is the first member of a category of drugs called alpha-glucosidase inhibitors. Acarbose slows down the time it takes for your intestine to break down food into glucose. This causes glucose to enter your blood more slowly. Your blood glucose then stays more even, with fewer highs and lows. Acarbose is especially helpful at flattening out the sharp rise in glucose that may occur after meals.

Possible side effects of acarbose

- Gas
- Bloating
- Diarrhea

Most people get these side effects when they first begin using acarbose. After a while, these side effects usually go away. But some people will still have the side effects. If you have any gastrointestinal diseases, do not take acarbose.

TROGLITAZONE

You may be prescribed troglitazone. It belongs to a class of drugs called thiazolidinediones. At this writing, troglitazone (brand name Rezulin) is approved for use in people with type 2 diabetes who are taking insulin. People with type 2 diabetes who take troglitazone may be able to reduce their insulin doses. Troglitazone enhances the action of insulin so that your body needs less. Troglitazone is not recommended for people with heart failure or liver disease.

PART OF THE DIABETES-CARE PLAN

Your doctor will tell you what pills to take, how many to take, and when to take them. Typically, you take them one to three times a day.

Oral agents do not take the place of diet and exercise. They work with diet and exercise. In fact, if you do not follow your meal and exercise plans, oral agents may not work for you.

Sometimes, oral agents work for a little while, then stop working. This often happens after several years. If your pills stop working, then your doctor may put you on

- Another pill
- Two different types of pills
- A pill and insulin
- Insulin

Pregnancy

Most women with diabetes have healthy babies. Often the biggest fear of women with diabetes is that their baby will get diabetes. In fact, the chances that their baby will get diabetes are small.

THE CHANCES THAT A BABY WILL GET DIABETES

If the mother has type 1 diabetes
   The baby has a 1 to 3 percent chance of getting diabetes.

If the father has type 1 diabetes
   The baby has a 3 to 6 percent chance of getting diabetes.

If either parent gets type 2 diabetes after age 50
   The baby has a 7 percent chance of getting diabetes.

If either parent gets type 2 diabetes before age 50
   The baby has a 14 percent chance of getting diabetes.

Although your baby may be safe from diabetes, there are other dangers to your baby's health and your own.

HIGH BLOOD GLUCOSE

One of the biggest dangers to you and your baby is high blood glucose levels. High blood glucose levels can lead to birth defects, macrosomia, and low blood glucose in your baby and to urinary tract infections in you.

Birth defects. High blood glucose levels during the first 8 weeks of your pregnancy can cause birth defects. It is during these early weeks that your baby's organs are forming.

Birth defects can affect any part of your baby. The heart, spinal cord, brain, and bones are most often affected. Because you have diabetes, birth defects are more likely to be severe and to cause miscarriages.

Macrosomia. Macrosomia means large body. If your blood glucose is too high during pregnancy, your baby may grow bigger and fatter than normal. This makes delivery harder. Babies who are larger than normal are more likely to have health problems.

Low blood glucose. High blood glucose levels right before or during labor can cause your baby to have low blood glucose after delivery.

Urinary tract infection. When your blood glucose is high during pregnancy, you are more likely to get a urinary tract infection. Urinary tract infections are usually caused by bacteria. Bacteria grow much better and faster in high glucose.

Signs of a urinary tract infection include the need to urinate often, pain or burning when you urinate, cloudy or bloody urine, low back pain or abdominal pain, fever, and chills.

HIGH KETONES

Ketones are made when your body burns stored fat for energy. Large amounts of ketones can harm you or your baby. Ketones are more likely to build up if you are not eating and drinking enough for both you and your baby. Be sure to eat all meals and snacks at your scheduled times.

DIABETES PILLS

Diabetes pills are not used during pregnancy because they may cause birth defects and low blood glucose in your baby. If you take diabetes pills, you will need to stop taking them before you get pregnant and while you are pregnant.

Your doctor may want to switch you to insulin. You may need insulin from early on in your pregnancy or just at the end of your pregnancy. Or you may not need any insulin at all.

PREECLAMPSIA

Preeclampsia (also called toxemia) is high blood pressure, swelling of your feet and lower legs, and leaking of protein into your urine during pregnancy. Other signs include headache, nausea, vomiting, abdominal pain, and blurred sight. If not treated, preeclampsia can cause seizures, coma, and death to you or your baby. Your doctor will watch for signs of preeclampsia.

HYDRAMNIOS

Hydramnios is excess amniotic fluid in your uterus. Signs of hydramnios are abdominal discomfort, larger-than-usual uterus, shortness of breath, and swelling of your legs. Hydramnios may cause premature labor. Your doctor will watch for signs of hydramnios.

TO INCREASE YOUR CHANCES OF A HEALTHY BABY

- *Get your blood glucose in good control before pregnancy.* If your blood glucose is in poor control, try to bring it into good control 3 to 6 months before you plan to get pregnant. If you wait until you know you are pregnant, your baby could already be harmed.

- *Keep your blood glucose in good control during your pregnancy.* This will require more frequent blood glucose testing. Staying in good control during your pregnancy can reduce the risk of problems for both you and your baby.

- *Test your urine for ketones every morning.* If you have moderate to large amounts of ketones in your urine, contact your doctor right away. You may need a change in diet or insulin.

- *Get fit before you get pregnant.* Exercising before pregnancy may increase your endurance, help lower your blood glucose, help you lose weight, and build up strength and flexibility.

- *Exercise during your pregnancy.* Pregnancy is not the time to start a vigorous exercise program, but you and your doctor can come up with exercises that are safe for you and your baby. Good exercises include walking, low-impact aerobics, swimming, and water aerobics.

- ***Follow your pregnancy meal plan.*** It is designed to help you avoid high and low blood glucose while providing what your baby needs to grow. Pregnancy is not the time to go on a weight-loss diet.

Sex and Diabetes

Diabetes and its complications can hurt your sex life. Sexual problems may have both physical and psychological causes. Doctors usually look for physical causes of sexual problems first.

PHYSICAL CAUSES

Too tired. If your blood glucose levels are high, you may feel too tired to have sex. Getting your diabetes under better control can help.

Urinary tract infection. When your blood glucose level is high, you are more likely to get a urinary tract infection. Signs of a urinary tract infection include:

- the need to urinate often
- pain or burning when you urinate
- cloudy or bloody urine
- low back pain or abdominal pain
- fever
- chills.

Sex may be painful or uncomfortable if you have a urinary tract infection. Urinary tract infections can be treated with antibiotic drugs.

Loss of sensation. If you have nerve damage, you may lose some sensation around your sex organs. This can make it harder for a woman to reach orgasm and for a man to get an erection. More intense direct stimulation of the sexual organs may help.

Lack of bladder control. If you have nerve damage to your bladder, you will not be able to tell when your bladder is full of urine. When you can't sense that your bladder is full, you are less likely to go to the bathroom. Not going to the bathroom often enough may cause you to dribble or wet yourself. This might happen during sex or orgasm. To prevent this, try emptying your bladder before and after sex.

Damaged limbs or joints. If you have nerve damage to a limb, are missing a limb, or have a joint disease, sex may be awkward or uncomfortable. Try different positions. Some may be better than others. Supporting yourself with several pillows may help. A physical therapist may be able to suggest ways for you to be more comfortable during sex.

Women only

Vaginal infection (vaginitis). Women with diabetes tend to get more vaginal infections than women without diabetes. Most vaginal infections are caused by the fungus *Candida albicans*. High blood glucose levels encourage the fungus to grow.

Signs of vaginitis include a thick white discharge, itching, burning, redness, and swelling. Vaginitis can cause irritation, discomfort, or pain during or after sex. Antifungal creams or drugs can clear up most vaginal infections. Getting your blood glucose under control may help prevent them.

Vaginal dryness. Vaginal dryness may be caused by nerve damage to the cells that line your vagina. Vaginal dryness can cause irritation, discomfort, or pain during or after sex.

Over-the-counter lubricants can help. Or your doctor can prescribe an estrogen vaginal cream. An estrogen vaginal cream adds wetness and helps rebuild damaged cells. Getting your blood glucose under control may delay or slow nerve damage.

Vaginal tightness (vaginismus). The pain or discomfort that you feel from vaginal infections or vaginal dryness can make you more likely to have vaginismus. Vaginismus is an involuntary spasm of the muscles around the vaginal entrance. It can make sex difficult or painful.

Learning to relax these muscles through Kegel exercises can help. In Kegel exercises, you tighten and release the same muscles you would use to stop the flow of urine. Try tensing and relaxing these muscles before or during sex. Or try positions in which you have more control over penetration.

If you have pain or discomfort during or after sex, see your doctor. Pain or discomfort can prevent orgasm and cause you to lose interest in sex.

Men only

Impotence. About half of men with diabetes become impotent. Impotence means that the penis does not become or stay hard enough for sex. There are many causes of impotence. The most common causes of impotence in men with diabetes are

- Damage to the nerves in your penis
- Damage to the blood vessels in your penis
- Poor control over your blood glucose levels

Physical impotence usually happens slowly and gets worse. Signs include a less rigid penis and fewer erections. Eventually, there are no erections. Keeping your blood glucose levels under control is the best way to avoid impotence. If you do become impotent, talk with your doctor. There are many treatment choices for physical impotence.

PSYCHOLOGICAL CAUSES

If you and your doctor have not been able to find a physical cause for your sexual problem, there may be a psychological cause. Psychological causes of sexual problems are the same whether you have diabetes or not. A sexual problem may be psychological if

- You are not able to talk with your partner about sex.
- You and your partner argue over money, children, work.
- You are stressed, worried, or anxious.
- You fear impotence.
- You fear pregnancy.

- You are sad, depressed, or angry.
- You had an inadequate sex education.
- You had a restrictive upbringing.
- You have been sexually abused.

If you think a psychological cause is a part of your sexual problem, seek out a mental health professional who specializes in this area. This might be a psychiatrist, psychologist, licensed social worker, or hypnotist.

Sick

Being sick with a cold or the flu can upset your diabetes-care plan. You may not be able to take your usual insulin or diabetes pills or to eat as you usually do. You may not even feel like eating. When you are sick, your blood glucose levels may go up too high or down too low.

To care for your diabetes when you are sick, make a plan for sick days. Your sick-day plan will help you know what medicines to take, what to eat and drink, how often to test, when to call your doctor, and what to tell your doctor. Your doctor and diabetes educator can help you make your sick-day plan.

WHAT MEDICINES TO TAKE

Most likely, you will keep taking your insulin or diabetes pills. You may even need extra.

If you have type 1 diabetes and your glucose levels are going up, your doctor may have you take extra Regular insulin to bring them down. If you have type 1 diabetes and have an upset stomach or don't feel like eating, you might take your long-acting insulin. If you use an insulin pump, you might adjust your usual dose.

If you control your diabetes with diet and exercise or with diabetes pills, you may need to take Regular insulin when you are sick. Your doctor may want you to keep a bottle of insulin on hand for sick days. Be sure you know how to give yourself an insulin shot before a sick day happens.

You may decide to take other kinds of medicines to care for your sickness. Some of these medicines may affect your blood glucose level. Decongestants and some cough syrups may raise your blood glucose level. Aspirin and some antibiotics may lower your blood glucose level. Ask your doctor or pharmacist whether the medicines you plan to take will affect your blood glucose levels.

WHAT TO EAT AND DRINK

Eat foods from your usual meal plan if you can. If you can't stick to your usual foods, follow your sick-day meal plan. It will include foods that are easy on your stomach. Try to eat a food with about 15 grams of carbohydrate in it every hour (see list of sick-day foods and fluids below). If you have a fever, are throwing up, or have diarrhea, you may lose too much fluid. Try to drink a cup of fluid each hour.

If your blood glucose level is over 240 mg/dl, drink sugar-free liquids like water, caffeine-free tea, sugar-free ginger ale, or broth (chicken, beef, or vegetable).

If your blood glucose level is less than 240 mg/dl, drink liquids with about 15 grams of carbohydrate in them (see list of sick-day foods and fluids below).

SICK-DAY FOODS AND FLUIDS
WITH ABOUT 15 GRAMS OF CARBOHYDRATE

6 saltine crackers	1/2 cup ice cream
5 vanilla wafers	1/2 cup cooked cereal
3 graham crackers	1/2 cup mashed potatoes
1 fruit juice bar	1/3 can regular soft drink
1 slice toast or bread	1/3 cup rice
1 cup soup	1/3 cup fruit-flavored yogurt
1 cup sports drink	1/4 cup applesauce
1/2 cup fruit juice	1/4 cup pudding
1/2 cup regular gelatin	1/4 cup sherbet

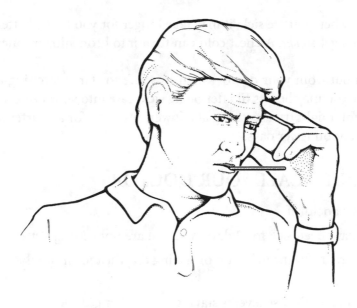

HOW OFTEN TO TEST

When you are sick, your body releases hormones that help it fight disease. These hormones can make your blood glucose level go up. They can also make it harder for your body to use insulin.

If you don't have enough insulin in your blood or you don't feel like eating, your body won't get the energy it needs. Your body may start to break down fat for energy. When your body breaks down fat, it makes waste products called ketones. Large amounts of ketones can harm you.

Your doctor will want you to test your blood glucose and urine ketones more often when you are sick. The sick-day plan you work out with your diabetes educator will tell you how often to test.

If you have type 1 diabetes, you may need to test your blood glucose and urine ketones every 3 to 4 hours. If you have type 2 diabetes, you may need to test your blood glucose four or five times a day and check your urine for ketones only if your glucose level is over 240 mg/dl.

HOW ABOUT EXERCISE?

Do not exercise when you are sick. Exercising when you are sick can make your blood glucose levels go down too low or up too high. If you exercise when you are sick, it may take longer for you to get better. You may even get sicker. A chest cold can turn into bronchitis or pneumonia.

Find out from your doctor when it is safe to start exercising again. Because you may be less fit after being sick, ease into your exercise program. You might try exercising at a lower intensity, for a shorter length of time, or on fewer days.

WHEN TO CALL YOUR DOCTOR

Call your doctor if

- You have been sick for 2 days, and you are not getting better.
- You have been throwing up or having diarrhea for more than 6 hours.
- Your blood glucose level is staying over 240 mg/dl.
- You have moderate or large amounts of ketones in your urine.
- You have any of these signs: chest pain, trouble breathing, fruity breath, or dry and cracked lips or tongue.
- You are not sure what to do to take care of yourself.

WHAT TO TELL YOUR DOCTOR

Keep written records so you can tell your doctor

- How long you have been sick
- What medicines you have taken and how much
- Whether you have been able to eat and drink
- How much you have been able to eat and drink
- Whether you are throwing up or having diarrhea
- Whether you have lost weight
- Your temperature
- Your blood glucose levels
- Your urine ketone levels

Skin Care

Diabetes makes skin problems more likely. Some skin problems are ones that anyone can have but that people with diabetes get more easily. These include bacterial infections and fungal infections. Other skin problems happen mostly to people with diabetes. These include diabetic dermopathy and digital sclerosis.

BACTERIAL INFECTIONS

Three bacterial infections that people with diabetes get more easily are styes, boils, and carbuncles. All three are most often caused by staphylococcal bacteria. All appear as red, painful, pus-filled lumps.

A stye is an infected gland of the eyelid. A boil is an infected hair root or skin gland. A carbuncle is a cluster of boils. Boils and carbuncles often occur at the back of your neck, armpits, groin, or buttocks.

If you think you have a stye, boil, carbuncle, or other bacterial infection, see your doctor.

FUNGAL INFECTIONS

Four fungal infections that people with diabetes get more easily are jock itch, athlete's foot, ringworm, and vaginal infections.

Jock itch is a red, itchy area that spreads from your genitals outward over the inside of your thighs. It is more common in men than women.

In athlete's foot, the skin between your toes becomes itchy and sore. It may crack and peel, or blister.

Ringworm is a ring-shaped, red, scaly patch that may itch or blister. It can appear on the feet, groin, scalp, nails, or trunk.

Vaginal infections are often caused by the fungus *Candida albicans*. It causes a thick white discharge from your vagina, and/or itching, burning, or irritation.

If you think you have a fungal infection, call your doctor.

DIABETIC DERMOPATHY

Diabetic dermopathy affects about 60 percent of men with diabetes who are over age 50 and 29 percent of women with diabetes who are over age 50.

It causes red or brown scaly patches on the front of your legs. Diabetic dermopathy is harmless and needs no treatment.

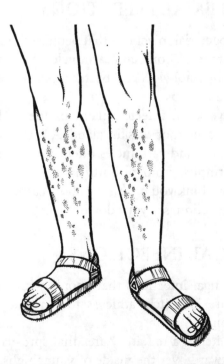

Diabetic dermopathy causes red or brown
patches on the front of your legs.

DIGITAL SCLEROSIS

Digital sclerosis affects up to 35 percent of people with diabetes. *Digital* refers to your fingers or toes. *Sclerosis* means hardening.

Digital sclerosis causes the skin on your hands, fingers, or toes to become thick and tight and look waxy or shiny. Sclerosis can cause aching and stiffness in your fingers.

Bringing blood glucose levels under control may slow or delay digital sclerosis. Pain killers and anti-inflammatory drugs can relieve aching joints.

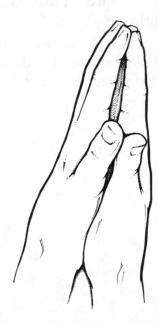

Digital sclerosis can make it hard to
press your fingers together.

TO KEEP YOUR SKIN HEALTHY

- *Keep your diabetes in good control.* High blood glucose levels make it easier for you to get bacterial and fungal infections. High blood glucose levels also tend to give you dry skin.

- *Keep your skin clean.* Take warm, not hot, baths or showers. Hot water can dry out your skin.

- *Keep dry parts of your skin moist.* Use moisturizers and moisturizing soaps. Keep your home more humid during cold, dry months. Drink plenty of water. It helps keep your skin moist, too.

- *Keep other parts of your skin dry.* Areas where skin touches skin need to be kept dry. These areas are between your toes, under your arms, and at your groin. Using powder on these areas can help keep them dry.

- *Protect your skin from the sun.* The sun can dry and burn your skin. When you are out in the sun, wear a waterproof, sweatproof sunscreen with an SPF (sun protection factor) of at least 15. Wearing a hat will also help.

- *Treat skin problems.* Over-the-counter products can be used to treat skin problems. But it's best to check with your doctor before using any skin treatment. And see a skin doctor (dermatologist) if skin problems don't go away.

Smoking

Quitting smoking is good for your diabetes. Quitting smoking is good for your health. When you quit smoking, you lower your blood glucose and blood pressure. You lower your total cholesterol, LDL cholesterol (the bad kind), and your triglycerides. When you quit smoking, you raise your HDL cholesterol (the good kind) and your oxygen intake. You even raise your life expectancy!

Quit smoking and you can reduce your risk for heart disease, blood vessel disease, kidney disease, nerve disease, dental disease, and cancer (mouth, throat, lungs, and bladder). You can reduce your risk of heart attack and stroke, miscarriage or stillbirth, limited joint mobility, and colds, bronchitis, and emphysema.

Quit smoking and you can even reduce your risk for insulin resistance (when your body does not respond to insulin). No wonder people try to quit. Here are some helpful hints.

BEFORE YOU QUIT

- Write down each time you smoke for a week. Write down any event or activity you were doing or about to do. Save the list.

- Write down all the reasons you want to quit. Read the list each day of the week before you quit.

- Pick a day to quit and write it down. Choose a day with few pressures. That way, stress won't tempt you to

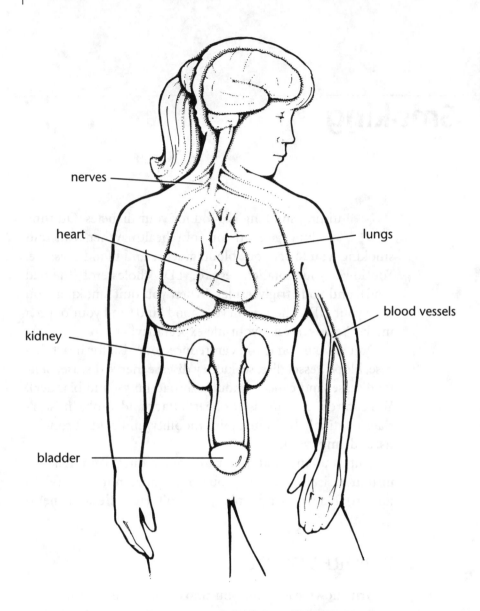

nerves

heart

lungs

blood vessels

kidney

bladder

Smoking can damage your heart, lungs, blood vessels, nerves, kidneys, and bladder. Smoking increases your risk of heart attack, stroke, miscarriages, and stillbirths.

smoke. You may want to do it when you've got some time off from work.

- Tell others you plan to quit. Let family, friends, and co-workers know. Seek their support. Tell them how they can help you. For example, ask them not to offer you a cigarette. Tell them what to expect when you first quit (see below).

- Choose a method of quitting. There are many ways to quit smoking. Not every method works for every person. Your diabetes-care team may be able to help you find a method that will work for you. It could be quitting "cold turkey." It might be using a nicotine patch or chewing gum. Hypnosis helps some people stop smoking. For others, acupuncture stops the craving to smoke.

- If you would find it easier to quit with other people, think about joining a stop-smoking class. Check for classes at local hospitals or local branches of organizations like the American Lung Association, the American Heart Association, and the American Cancer Society.

- Practice deep breathing. Relaxation tapes may help.

- Stock up on raw vegetables and other low-fat, low-calorie snacks. Your appetite may increase after you quit smoking. You may gain weight (the average gain is 7 pounds). You may crave sweet foods.

- Begin to exercise a few weeks before you quit smoking. More activity will help you combat withdrawal symptoms and weight gain. Exercise can take the place of smoking or help you control the urge to eat. Try brisk walking, cycling, or swimming.

- Plan rewards for not smoking. For example, you might play a favorite game one week, go to a movie the next week.

WHEN YOU QUIT

You may go through withdrawal for a few days or weeks. The table on the next page lists some of the symptoms you may feel and how to deal with them.

AFTER YOU QUIT

The first 3 months or so after quitting are the hardest. Most people who return to smoking do so then. Try these tactics for staying smoke-free.

- Refer to the list you made of events or activities that were going on around the time you smoked. The next time any of those events or activities comes up, avoid it. For example, if you always smoke at happy hour, don't go.

    If you can't avoid the event, replace the cigarette with something else. Hold something else in your hand. Try a strand of beads, a polished stone, or a pen. Put something else in your mouth, like a toothpick. Chew gum or ice.

- If you smoke to relax, find another way to relax. Try deep breathing or relaxation exercises. If you smoke to perk up, try a walk or stretching.

- Throw away your cigarettes, butts, lighters, matches, and ashtrays.

- Put your list of reasons for quitting where you had kept your cigarettes.

- Read your list of reasons for quitting. Remind yourself that you don't want to smoke.

- Remind yourself that all it takes is one cigarette to become a smoker again. Try to avoid even one.

- Make a list of things you like about not smoking.

- If you are worried about gaining weight, talk with your dietitian about changing your meal and exercise plans.

WITHDRAWAL

Symptom	Duration	Solution
Urge to smoke	Strong first 2 weeks, then on and off	Do something else.
Blood glucose goes up and down	Varies	Monitor closely.
Irritable, tense, on edge	Several weeks	Take a break or a walk. Listen to a relaxation tape.
Trouble concentrating or feel "out of it"	Several weeks	Break up big tasks into smaller ones. Take short breaks.
Extra energy or restlessness	Varies	Exercise.
Sleepy during the day	2 to 4 weeks	Take a walk or a nap.
Trouble sleeping at night	Less than 7 days	Try deep breathing. Avoid caffeine after 5 p.m.
Constipation	3 to 4 weeks	Add fiber (raw fruits, vegetables, whole-grain breads and cereals) to diet. Drink 6 to 8 glasses of water a day.
Coughing	Less than 7 days	Sip water.
Headache, muscle cramps, nausea, or sweating	Few days	Try a warm bath or some quiet time.
Craving sweets	Several weeks	Eat a low-calorie snack.

Snacks

Snacks are usually included as part of your meal plan if you take insulin or diabetes pills. Eating snacks helps you keep your blood glucose from going too low.

Your dietitian will give you ideas for snacks and snack times. A healthy snack is a food that contains about 15 grams of carbohydrate.

HEALTHY SNACKS

6 crackers with low-fat cheese

3 pieces of dried fruit

2 fig bars

2 oatmeal-raisin cookies

1 cup of soup

1/2 cup of cereal

1/2 cup of fruit juice

1/2 bagel

1/2 pita

1/2 cup of pasta

1 slice of bread with a slice of turkey breast

1 slice of bread with reduced-fat peanut butter

1 English muffin

1 cup of low-fat or nonfat fruit yogurt

2 bread sticks

2 rice cakes

1 granola bar

1 piece of fruit

1 small roll

1 tortilla

1/3 cup of baked beans

There are times when you might need extra snacks or times when you need to be careful not to forget your snacks.

EXERCISE

You might need to eat extra snacks before, during, or after exercise. Test your blood glucose 30 minutes before exercise and again just before you begin. If the tests show that your blood glucose is dropping, you may need to eat an extra snack before you start.

If you will be exercising for more than 1 hour, you will need to eat snacks for every 30 minutes of exercise. After exercise, blood glucose levels may keep falling for as long as 10 to 24 hours. Test your blood glucose during this time. If tests show that your blood glucose is dropping too low, you may need an extra snack after exercise.

NEW BABY

When you have a new baby to care for, it is easy to lose track of your scheduled snacks and meals. You can be so busy you forget to eat. Or you can be so tired you sleep right through a snack or mealtime. You'll need to be careful of low blood glucose, especially if you have type 1 diabetes. Be sure to eat your regular snacks and meals. And don't nap or go to sleep with an empty stomach.

BREAST-FEEDING

Breast-feeding uses up many calories and nutrients. Snacking gives needed nutrients and calories back to your body and helps prevent low blood glucose.

During the day, eat your snack (or meal) before breast-feeding or while you are breast-feeding. It helps to have the snack or meal ready ahead of time. Have a snack during night feedings, too. If you don't, you are likely to have low blood glucose the next morning.

Stress

Our lives are full of things that can cause stress. Stress can be physical, like an injury or an illness. Stress can be mental, like problems with your job, marriage, or finances. Some stresses can be good, like those that gear you up for a competition. But good or bad, any stress that lasts a long time can wear your body down. Diabetes is a physical stress that lasts a long time. Having to take care of your diabetes can make you feel stressed.

When you feel stressed, your body gets ready for action. It pumps stress hormones into your blood. Stress hormones make your body release stored glucose and stored fat for extra energy. This extra energy helps your body face up to or run away from the stress. But the extra glucose and fat can only be used by your body if there is enough insulin.

In people with diabetes, there may not be enough insulin. And the stress hormones themselves may make it harder for your body to use the insulin that is there. When there is not enough insulin, glucose and fat build up in the blood. This can lead to high glucose levels and high ketones.

To avoid high glucose and high ketones, you need to know what happens to your blood glucose levels when you are under stress. The type of stress you are under may make a difference. Physical stress causes blood glucose levels to go up in most people with diabetes. Mental stress causes some people's glucose levels to go up and other people's glucose levels to go down. To see which way your blood glucose goes, try the following test.

BLOOD GLUCOSE STRESS TEST

Before you test your blood glucose, rate your level of stress. You can use a number from 1 to 10 or the words *high, medium,* or *low.* Write down your stress rating. Now test your blood glucose. Record your blood glucose test results. Do this for a week or two.

Compare the blood glucose test results with your stress ratings. Does high blood glucose occur with high stress? If so, you may need more insulin when you are under stress. Check with your doctor first.

TO HANDLE STRESS

1. Make a list of things that stress you. Each one of us is different. What causes little or no stress for you may cause great stress for somebody else. This list of stressors may get you started:

Job	Unemployment	Retirement
Illness	Elderly parents	Grief
Divorce	In-Laws	Separation
Children	Holidays	Travel
Traffic	Car trouble	Moving

2. Learn how you react to stress. Pay attention to how you feel. How you feel may be different from what someone else feels. You may feel tense, anxious, upset, or angry. You may feel tired, sad, or empty. Your stomach or head may hurt.

3. Change how you react to stress. Often you can't stop things that cause stress. But you can change how you react. If you feel stressed, try some of the tactics listed below. Find the ones that work best for you.

TO REDUCE STRESS

Breathe deeply . Sit or lie down. Close your eyes. Breathe in deeply and slowly. Let all the breath out. Breathe in and out again.

Start to relax your muscles. Keep breathing in and out. Each time you breathe out, relax your muscles even more. Do this for 5 to 20 minutes. Do it at least once a day.

Let go. Lie down. Close your eyes. Tense and release the muscles of each body part. Start at your head, and work your way down to your feet.

Loosen up. Circle, stretch, and shake parts of your body.

Get a massage. Put yourself in the hands of a licensed massage therapist.

Think good thoughts. Your thoughts affect your feelings. Put a rubber band on your wrist. Snap it each time you think a bad thought. Replace that bad thought with a better thought. Or repeat a happy poem, prayer, or quote.

Talk about it. Talk about your troubles. It may help you feel better. Confide in family or friends. Consult a therapist or join a support group. Others may be having the same troubles you are.

Put it on paper. Write down what's bothering you. You may find a solution. Or draw or paint your worries away.

Try something new. Start a hobby or learn a craft. Take a class. Join a club or a team. Volunteer at a school, hospital, church, charity, or other community organization. Go away for the weekend.

Stay active. Some of the best activities for relieving stress are circuit training, cross-country skiing, bicycling, rowing, running, and swimming. If you don't like any of these, choose an activity you like, and do it often.

Listen up. Listen to music you find soothing. Or play a tape of nature sounds, like birds or ocean waves.

Soak in a warm bath. The most comfortable bath water is about the same temperature as your skin. Probably between 85° and 93°F. Linger in the bath for 20 to 30 minutes. Add bubbles or soothing herbs if you like.

Learn to say no. Especially, don't do things you really don't want to do. You may feel stressed if you take on too much.

Laugh about it. Have a hearty healthy laugh. Seek out funny movies, funny books, and funny people.

Look at nature. Look at the world around you—flowers, trees, even bugs. The sun, the moon, the stars. Clouds, wind, and rain. Just go outside and spend time there. If you can't go outside, look out a window. Even looking at pictures of nature can help you slow down and relax.

Eat wisely. When you are under stress, your body may use up more B vitamins, vitamin C, protein, and calcium.

Replenish your B vitamins by eating more whole grains, nuts, seeds, and beans. Boost your vitamin C with oranges, grapefruits, and broccoli. Beef up your protein with chicken, fish, and egg whites. Stock up your calcium with low-fat milk, yogurt, and cheese.

Sleep on it. Sometimes things look better the next day. Get your 7 to 9 hours of sleep a day.

Stroke

A stroke occurs when blood flow to the brain is blocked. Without blood, the brain can't get the oxygen it needs. Part of the brain gets damaged or dies.

Blood flow can be cut off by a buildup of fat and cholesterol in the blood vessels that lead to the brain (see Blood Vessel Disease). This type of stroke is called an ischemic stroke. It is the most common type.

If blood flow to the brain is blocked for only a brief time, it is called a transient ischemic attack (TIA). Your body may release enzymes that dissolve the clot quickly and restore blood flow. If you have TIAs often, you are more likely to have an ischemic stroke.

Another type of stroke is a hemorrhagic stroke. It occurs when a blood vessel in your brain leaks or breaks. The most common cause of hemorrhagic strokes is high blood pressure. High blood pressure can weaken blood vessels. Weak blood vessels are more likely to leak or break.

Having diabetes doubles your chances of having a stroke. If you have other risk factors for stroke, your chances of having a stroke are even greater.

RISK FACTORS FOR STROKE

- You have had TIAs.
- You have had high blood pressure.
- You smoke.
- You have high cholesterol.

- You are overweight.
- You do not exercise.
- You drink too much alcohol.

You can't change the fact that you have diabetes. But you can reduce your other risk factors.

TO REDUCE YOUR RISK OF STROKE

- If your diabetes is in poor control, try to keep your blood glucose levels in your ideal range (see Blood Glucose). This may prevent or delay blood vessel damage caused by high blood glucose.
- If you have high blood pressure, work with your doctor to control it. You can bring your blood pressure down with a healthy diet, exercise, weight loss, and blood pressure drugs. Cutting down on sodium (salt) lowers blood pressure for some people. Aim for less than 2,000 milligrams of sodium a day.
- If you smoke, try to cut down or quit. Smoking narrows blood vessels and promotes the buildup of fat and cholesterol on blood vessel walls. Smoking makes blood clot faster.
- If you have high cholesterol, eat less saturated animal fats and cholesterol. High cholesterol can damage blood vessels.
- If you are overweight, lose a few pounds! Losing even a little weight with diet and exercise lowers blood pressure and improves cholesterol levels.
- If you don't exercise, try walking or biking for as little as 15 minutes three times a week! These types of aerobic exercise can lower your blood pressure, lower your LDL (bad) cholesterol and triglycerides, and raise your HDL (good) cholesterol.
- If you drink more than two drinks a day, cut back. Drinking that much alcohol can raise your blood pressure. Drink no more than 2 ounces of liquor, 2 glasses of wine, or 2 beers a day. Don't drink at all if you have a drinking problem or a medical reason not to drink.

Be alert to the warning signs of stroke. Know what to do if the warning signs occur.

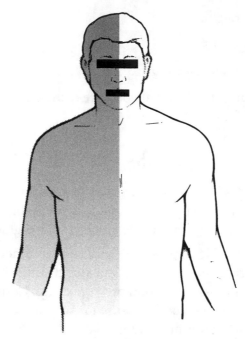

A stroke can cause difficulty seeing or talking or lead to weakness on one side of your body.

WARNING SIGNS OF A STROKE OR TIA

- You are suddenly weak or numb in your face, an arm, or a leg.
- Your sight is suddenly dim, blurred, or lost.
- You can't speak or can't understand someone else who is talking.
- You have a sudden headache.
- You feel dizzy or unsteady, or you suddenly fall.

IF YOU THINK YOU ARE HAVING A STROKE

1. Call 911 for an ambulance.
2. Remain calm.
3. Do not eat or drink anything.

Sugars

Sugars are one of the two major types of carbohydrate. The other major type is starch. Sugars and starches are broken down into glucose by your body. Sugars and starches raise your blood glucose level.

Research has shown that sugars do not raise your blood glucose level any more than starches or other carbohydrates. Because of these findings, the American Diabetes Association allows sugars in a diabetes meal plan.

Sugars can be part of your total carbohydrate for the day. You and your dietitian can figure out how to fit sugars into your meal plan so they will not hurt your blood glucose control.

WHERE THE SUGARS ARE

Sugars occur naturally in fruits, vegetables, and dairy products. Foods with natural sugars are usually good sources of nutrients, such as vitamins, minerals, fiber, and protein.

Sugars may be added to foods during processing. You can find out how many sugars a food has by reading the Nutrition Facts on food labels (see Food Labeling).

Many nutritious foods, such as breakfast cereals, breads, and low-fat salad dressings, contain some added sugars. Other foods with added sugar, such as chocolate, baked goods, and ice cream treats, provide lots of calories and fat with few nutrients. If you are trying to lose weight, you will want to limit sugary, high-calorie, high-fat foods.

KINDS OF SUGARS

There are many kinds of sugars. The ingredients list on a food label may tell you the kinds of sugars in a food. Here's a list of names of sugars or foods that are made mostly of sugars:

Dextrose	Beet sugar	Carob powder
Fructose	Brown sugar	Cornstarch
Galactose	Cane sugar	Corn sweetener
Glucose	Confectioner's sugar	Corn syrup
Lactose	Granulated sugar	Honey
Levulose	Invert sugar	Maple syrup
Maltose	Maple sugar	Molasses
Sucrose	Powdered sugar	Starch syrup
Sorghum	Raw sugar	Sugar cane syrup
Turbinado	Table sugar	

THE CALORIES IN SUGARS

The sugars listed above average about 16 calories per teaspoon. Some, like powdered sugar (10 calories) and fructose (12 calories), are lower in calories. Others, like honey (21 calories) and molasses (18 calories), are higher in calories.

Sugar alcohols, which may be added to foods, have fewer calories than sugars. Sugar alcohols include sorbitol, xylitol, isomalt, lactitol, hydrogenated starch hydrolysates, mannitol, and maltitol.

The calories in sugars can be a source of energy for people who are very physically active. Very active people burn lots of calories and have higher calorie needs. If you don't exercise and do very little other physical activity, you probably need fewer calories. Your dietitian may ask you to go easy on sugary foods. If you spend your daily amount of calories on sugary foods, you may not have much left for your meals.

FRUCTOSE AND THE SUGAR ALCOHOLS

Fructose and the sugar alcohols may cause a smaller rise in your blood glucose level than other sugars or starches. But large amounts of fructose may increase your blood fat levels. And large amounts of sugar alcohols may give you diarrhea.

The American Diabetes Association recommends that people use foods sweetened with fructose or the sugar alcohols in moderate amounts. There is no reason to use large amounts of fructose or the sugar alcohols in place of other sugars.

NONNUTRITIVE SWEETENERS

Nonnutritive sweeteners have very few calories and will not affect your blood glucose level. Unlike sugars, they can be added to your meal plan. The American Diabetes Association approves the use of three nonnutritive sweeteners in moderate amounts. These are aspartame (Nutrasweet, Equal), saccharin (Sweet'n Low), and acesulfame potassium (Sweet One).

THE CHOICE IS YOURS

Whether you choose to use sugars, nonnutritive sweeteners, or both is up to you and your dietitian. The American Dietetic Association recommends that all people use added sugars and other sweeteners in moderation as part of a nutritious and well-balanced diet.

Type 1 Diabetes

n type 1 diabetes, your body stops making insulin or makes only a tiny amount. When this happens, you need to take insulin to live and to be healthy.

Without insulin, glucose cannot get into your cells. Your cells need glucose to burn for energy. Glucose collects in the blood. Over time, high levels of glucose in the blood may hurt your eyes, kidneys, nerves, or heart.

Type 1 diabetes occurs most often in people under age 30 years. But it can occur at any age. The signs of type 1 diabetes can come on suddenly and be severe.

SIGNS OF TYPE 1 DIABETES

Frequent urination	Fatigue
Constant hunger	Edginess
Constant thirst	Mood changes
Weight loss	Nausea
Weakness	Vomiting

CAUSES OF TYPE 1 DIABETES

No one knows for sure why people get type 1 diabetes. Some people are born with genes that make them more likely to get it. But many other people with the same genes do not get diabetes. Something else inside or outside the body triggers the disease. Experts don't know what that something is yet. But they are trying to find out.

Most people with type 1 diabetes have high levels of autoantibodies in their blood sometime before they are first diagnosed with the disease. Antibodies are proteins your body makes to destroy germs or viruses. Autoantibodies are antibodies that have "gone bad." They attack your body's own tissues. In people who get type 1 diabetes, autoantibodies may attack insulin or the cells that make insulin.

TREATMENT FOR TYPE 1 DIABETES

There is no cure for diabetes. But there are things you can do to care for type 1 diabetes. The things you do to care for your diabetes help you bring blood glucose levels within your ideal range.

1. Take insulin. Insulin shots or an insulin pump replaces the insulin you no longer make. Insulin lets your cells take in glucose.
2. Follow a healthy meal plan (see Meal Planning).
3. Stay physically active. Being active helps your cells take in glucose.
4. Do blood tests. Self-tests help you track how well you are doing.
5. Get regular checkups. Your doctor can help you make changes in your diabetes-care plan.

BRITTLE DIABETES

Brittle diabetes refers to wide, unpredictable swings in blood glucose. Now that blood glucose monitoring is possible for everyone, people can usually get a good idea of what their blood glucose level is going to do. Why do some people's blood glucose levels swing so wide? Because their bodies have exaggerated responses to food, medication, and stress. Food is not absorbed in the same amount of time every time you eat. Insulin is absorbed at different rates. The stresses and strains of everyday living create the release of different amounts of stress hormones at different times. These work alone or together to produce the wide swings in blood glucose levels.

If you have brittle diabetes, work with your health care provider on your insulin injection dose, technique, sites, depth, and timing. You may need to keep careful records for awhile until you get enough clues to figure out what is causing those extreme highs and lows.

Type 2 Diabetes

In type 2 diabetes, your body does not make enough insulin, or your body has trouble using the insulin, or both. A person with type 2 diabetes might inject insulin but does not depend on it to live.

Without enough insulin, your cells cannot use the glucose in your blood to make energy. Instead, glucose stays in the blood. This can lead to high blood glucose levels. Over time, high blood glucose levels may hurt your eyes, kidneys, nerves, or heart.

Most people who get type 2 diabetes are over 40 years old. But it may occur in younger people.

SIGNS OF TYPE 2 DIABETES

Frequent urination	Tingling or numb hands or feet
Constant thirst	
Constant hunger	Fatigue
Weight loss	Weakness
Dry, itchy skin	Infections of the skin, gums, bladder, or vagina that keep
Blurred vision	coming back or heal slowly

CAUSES OF TYPE 2 DIABETES

Doctors don't know for sure what causes type 2 diabetes. They do know that type 2 diabetes runs in families. If other members of your family have type 2 diabetes, you are much more likely to get it. But it usually takes something else to bring on the disease. For many people with diabetes, being overweight brings it on. type 2 diabetes is common in people who

- Eat too much fat
- Eat too little carbohydrate and fiber
- Get too little exercise

Such habits can make you overweight. When you are overweight, your body has a harder time using the insulin that it makes. This is called insulin resistance. In insulin resistance, your body does not respond to insulin as it should.

TREATMENT OF TYPE 2 DIABETES

There is no cure for diabetes. But there are ways to lower your blood glucose levels and improve your body's use of insulin.

At first, diet and exercise may work. Through diet and exercise, you may lose weight. Losing weight can help some people get their blood glucose into a more normal range. Diet and exercise help your body use the insulin you have. If diet and exercise do not control your blood glucose, you may need diabetes pills.

Diabetes pills are drugs that lower blood glucose levels. They are not insulin. If diet, exercise, and diabetes pills do not lower blood glucose, you may need to add insulin. Or insulin may replace the diabetes pills.

TO CARE FOR YOUR DIABETES

- Eat healthy foods.
- Control your weight.
- Stay physically active.
- Take diabetes pills or insulin, if needed.
- Test your blood glucose.
- Get regular checkups.

Vegetarian Diets

Avegetarian diet is based on plant foods. Plant foods include fruits, vegetables, grains, legumes (beans, peas, and lentils), nuts, and seeds. Plant foods have no cholesterol. Most are low in fat and calories. All are high in fiber, vitamins, and minerals.

A vegetarian diet can be a healthy choice for people with diabetes. Vegetarians are less likely to be overweight, to have high cholesterol levels, or to have high blood pressure. Vegetarians are less likely to get heart disease, blood vessel disease, colon or lung cancer, or osteoporosis.

People with type 1 diabetes who become vegetarians may need less insulin. People with type 2 diabetes who become vegetarians may lose weight. Losing weight may improve blood glucose control.

Many people who think about eating a vegetarian diet wonder if they will get enough protein. But there is little need to worry.

Most vegetarians are able to get all the protein they need from high-protein grains, legumes, nuts, and seeds. Other vegetarians also get protein from certain animal foods, such as low-fat dairy products, fish, shellfish, and poultry.

Whether a vegetarian eats animal foods depends on the kind of vegetarian he or she is. There are five kinds of vegetarians: vegan, lactovegetarian, ovovegetarian, lactoovovegetarian, and semivegetarian. See the tables that follow to find out what each kind of vegetarian eats and how much food a vegetarian should eat.

WHAT A VEGETARIAN EATS

Type	Eats	Does Not Eat
Vegan	Fruits, vegetables, legumes, grains, nuts, seeds	Meat, fish, shellfish, poultry, dairy products, eggs
Lacto-vegetarian	Fruits, vegetables, legumes, grains, nuts, seeds, dairy products	Meat, fish, shellfish, poultry, eggs
Ovo-vegetarian	Fruits, vegetables, legumes, grains, nuts, seeds, eggs	Meat, fish, shellfish, poultry, dairy products
Lactoovo-vegetarian	Fruits, vegetables, legumes, grains, nuts, seeds, eggs, dairy products	Meat, fish, shellfish, poultry
Semi-vegetarian	Fruits, vegetables, legumes, grains, nuts, seeds, eggs, dairy products, fish, shellfish, poultry	Meat

HOW MUCH A VEGETARIAN MIGHT EAT

Food	Servings Per Day
Grains	6 to 11
Vegetables	3 to 8
Fruits	2 to 4
Legumes	2 to 3
Dairy products	2 to 4
Nuts and seeds	1 to 2
Fats and oils	1 to 2

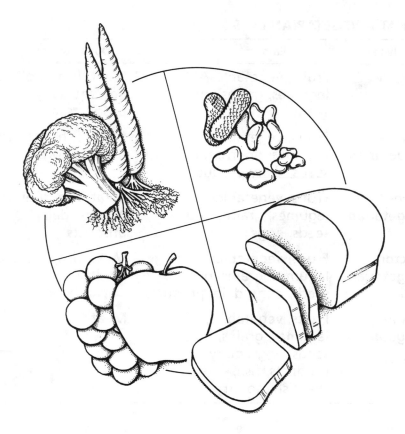

A healthy diet contains foods from different groups.

If you would like to try a vegetarian diet, talk with a dietitian. A dietitian can help you substitute foods for those you want to take out of your meal plan. A dietitian can help you make sure you get all the nutrients—vitamins, minerals, protein, fats, and carbohydrates—that your body needs. Here are a few suggestions for "going vegetarian."

GOING VEGETARIAN

- Start by eating one vegetarian meal a week for several weeks. Stick with familiar foods at first, like spaghetti with marinara sauce.

- Read vegetarian cookbooks for recipe ideas.
- Try eating out at a vegetarian restaurant. You may be surprised by the variety of tasty dishes you'll find.
- Eat less meat, poultry, fish, and shellfish in your meals. An ideal portion is 3 ounces—about the size of a deck of cards.
- Cut meat into cubes or strips and add to a salad or grain dish.
- Eat more grains, legumes, and vegetables in your meals.
- Try cooked beans in place of some of the meat in your chili, stir-fries, stews, and casseroles.

Vitamins and Minerals

The right amounts of vitamins and minerals help your body function well. You can get vitamins and minerals from the foods you eat. You can also get vitamins and minerals from pills. These are called supplements.

Most people with diabetes get enough vitamins and minerals by eating a variety of foods. Some people with diabetes may be deficient in certain vitamins and minerals. Being deficient means your body does not have enough of a vitamin or mineral.

VITAMIN DEFICIENCIES

Most people with diabetes get enough vitamin A. Most people with diabetes also get enough vitamin E and vitamin C, but a few people may need more. Check with your doctor about this.

People with diabetes usually get enough of the B vitamins. The B vitamins include vitamin B_1 (thiamin), vitamin B_2 (riboflavin), vitamin B_3 (niacin), vitamin B_6 (pyridoxine), vitamin B_{12}, and folate. If your diabetes is in poor control, though, you risk losing the B vitamins in your urine. Your doctor may advise you to eat more foods high in the B vitamins.

Research has shown that a deficiency in vitamin B_6 may be related to impaired glucose tolerance. Impaired glucose tolerance means your body has a hard time using insulin.

FOOD SOURCES OF VITAMINS AND MINERALS

Vitamin A	Liver, tuna, deep-orange fruits and vegetables, leafy greens
Vitamin B_1 (thiamin)	Pork, sunflower seeds, whole grains
Vitamin B_2 (riboflavin)	Liver, duck, mackerel, dairy foods
Vitamin B_3 (niacin)	Poultry, fish, veal
Vitamin B_6 (pyridoxine)	Potatoes, bananas, chickpeas, prune juice, poultry, fish, liver
Vitamin B_{12}	Fish, shellfish, liver
Vitamin C	Citrus fruits, melon, strawberries, kiwifruit, bell peppers, broccoli, Brussels sprouts
Vitamin D	Fish, fortified milk, butter, margarine, eggs
Vitamin E	Nuts, seeds, oils, mangos, blackberries, apples
Folate	Legumes, leafy greens, asparagus, liver, wheat germ
Calcium	Yogurt, milk, cheese
Chromium	Wheat germ, brewer's yeast, bran, whole grains, liver, meats, cheese
Copper	Crab, liver, nuts, seeds, prunes, raisins
Iron	Shellfish, meats, liver, soybeans, pumpkin seeds
Magnesium	seeds, legumes, whole grains, leafy greens, fish
Manganese	Whole grains, vegetables, nuts, fruits
Potassium	Fruits, vegetables, legumes, fish, milk, yogurt
Selenium	Shellfish, fish, liver, nuts, whole grains
Zinc	Meats, liver, shellfish

MINERAL DEFICIENCIES

Most people with diabetes get enough chromium. But a few people with diabetes have a chromium deficiency. A chromium deficiency can cause higher blood glucose and blood fat levels and impaired glucose tolerance.

If a lab test shows that you have a chromium deficiency, your doctor may have you take a chromium supplement. If you already get enough chromium, taking extra will not help your blood glucose or blood fat levels.

Deficiencies in copper and manganese have been linked to impaired glucose tolerance. But most people with diabetes get enough copper and manganese. So deficiencies are not likely. Deficiencies in selenium are not likely either. And most people with diabetes are not at any greater risk for iron deficiency than people without diabetes.

People with diabetes who have poor blood glucose control or have very high ketones are more likely to become deficient in magnesium. A lack of magnesium may make your body less sensitive to insulin. If a lab test shows that your magnesium level is low, your doctor may have you take magnesium supplements.

Deficiencies in zinc are more likely in people with diabetes, especially those in poor control. Lack of zinc may cause impaired glucose tolerance. If a lab test shows you do not have enough zinc, your doctor may have you take a supplement or eat more foods high in zinc.

VITAMIN OR MINERAL SUPPLEMENTS

Check with your doctor or dietitian to be sure you are getting the vitamins and minerals you need. If your doctor or dietitian finds that you lack some vitamins and minerals, he or she may recommend a supplement.

If you are dieting and take in fewer than 1,200 calories each day
   You may need iron and folate.

If you eat no animal foods at all
   You may need vitamin B_{12}, calcium, iron, vitamin B_2 (riboflavin), and zinc.

If you are at risk for bone diseases
You may need vitamin D, calcium, and magnesium.

If you are over 65
You may need calcium and folate.

If you are pregnant or breast-feeding
You may need extra iron, zinc, calcium, and folate.

If you take diuretics (water pills)
You may need magnesium, calcium, potassium, and zinc.

Check with your doctor before taking any supplement.

THE RIGHT DOSE

The National Academy of Sciences establishes Recommended Dietary Allowances (RDAs) and Safe and Adequate Intakes for vitamins and minerals. These are the minimum amounts of vitamins and minerals that most people need. Healthy people with diabetes need to get these amounts.

RECOMMENDED DIETARY ALLOWANCES OR SAFE AND ADEQUATE INTAKES OF VITAMINS AND MINERALS FOR MEN AND WOMEN AGED 25 TO 50 YEARS

	Men	Women
Vitamin A	1,000 µg RE	800 µg RE
Vitamin B_1 (thiamin)	1.5 mg	1.1 mg
Vitamin B_2 (riboflavin)	1.7 mg	1.3 mg
Vitamin B_3 (niacin)	19 mg	15 mg
Vitamin B_6 (pyridoxine)	2 mg	1.6 mg
Vitamin B_{12}	2.0 µg	2.0 µg
Vitamin C	60 mg	60 mg
Vitamin D	5 µg	5 µg
Vitamin E	10 mg aTE	8 mg aTE
Folate	200 µg	180 µg
Calcium	800 mg	800 mg
Chromium	50 to 200 µg	50 to 200 µg
Copper	1.5 to 3.0 mg	1.5 to 3.0 mg
Iron	10 mg	15 mg
Magnesium	350 mg	280 mg
Manganese	2.0 to 5.0 mg	2.0 to 5.0 mg
Potassium	3,500 mg	3,500 mg
Selenium	70 µg	55 µg
Zinc	15 mg	12 mg

RE stands for retinol equivalents. Since 1974, the National Academy of Sciences has been using retinol equivalents (RE) instead of international units (I.U.) to measure vitamin A in food for vitamin A requirements. aTE stands for alpha-tocopherol equivalents. Alpha-tocopherol is the most easily absorbed form of vitamin E.

Weight Loss

If you are overweight, losing weight is one of the best treatments for type 2 diabetes. Losing weight will lower your blood pressure, lower your risk of heart disease and blood vessel disease, and improve your blood glucose control.

Your blood glucose control may improve so much that you can stop taking or cut down on your insulin or diabetes pills. Sometimes, losing just 10 to 20 pounds is enough to improve diabetes control, even if that does not get you to your ideal body weight.

To find your ideal body weight, measure your height. Women, count your first 5 feet as 100 pounds, and add 5 pounds for each inch over 5 feet. Men, count your first 5 feet as 106 pounds, and add 6 pounds for each inch over 5 feet.

Your answer is your ideal body weight, if you have a medium frame. If you have a small frame, subtract 10%. If you have a large frame, add 10%. You are overweight if you are 30% above your ideal body weight.

If you are overweight, check with your health care team about how much weight loss would be good for you. Set a weight-loss goal. Break down your goal into smaller goals that you can easily meet. You may set weekly or monthly weight-loss goals.

When you meet a smaller goal, reward yourself with a book, a CD, an outing, or a piece of clothing, for example. Once you have set your goals, you are ready to start your weight-loss program.

The only way to lose weight is to eat less and exercise more. The only way to keep the weight off is to keep up these two new habits even after you have lost the weight.

EAT LESS

Eating less actually means eating fewer calories. To do this, you may need to eat smaller portions. Or, you may be able to eat the same amount of food, if you eat foods that are lower in calories.

Fat has more than twice as many calories as carbohydrate or protein. So if you eat less fat and eat more carbohydrates and protein, you will get fewer calories.

To eat less fat, try low-fat or nonfat versions of your favorite high-fat foods. Grill, broil, bake, steam, or poach your food instead of frying it. Eat less butter, margarine, oil, sauces, and gravy. And limit high-calorie, low-nutrient foods like desserts, soft drinks, and chips.

To get more carbohydrates, choose high-fiber foods. High-fiber foods include fruits, vegetables, and whole-grain breads, cereals, and pastas. For more protein, choose beans, lean meat, fish, and poultry without the skin.

Dieting tips

- Serve food from the kitchen. And leave it there instead of putting it on the table. Going for seconds won't be as easy.
- Eat slowly and stop when you are just full, not too full.
- Don't watch TV, read, or listen to the radio while you eat. These activities may draw your attention away from how much you are eating.
- Brush your teeth right after you eat. This gets the taste of food out of your mouth and may get the thought of food out of your head.
- Don't go grocery shopping when you are hungry. You may buy too much.
- Store food out of sight.

- Eat something before you go to a social function. That way, you'll be less likely to overeat fatty foods.

- Don't skip a meal. You may overeat at your next one.

- Don't forbid yourself to eat certain foods. You'll only want them more. Try to cut down on portion sizes or the number of times you eat those foods.

EXERCISE MORE

Exercise takes weight off by helping you burn more calories than you take in. If you exercise regularly, your muscles will burn calories even while you're at rest.

Different exercises burn different numbers of calories. Some good exercises for weight loss are cross-country skiing, brisk walking, fast swimming, bicycling, and low-impact aerobics.

It's best to exercise at a moderate pace for a long time. If you exercise at a high pace, you will tire yourself out before you have a chance to burn enough calories.

The longer you exercise, the more calories you burn. Build up to where you can do an aerobic type of exercise for 45 to 60 minutes, four or more times a week.

To burn even more calories, add physical activities throughout the day. Walk, don't drive. Take the stairs, not the elevator. Play with the kids. Work in your garden. Spend the night out bowling or dancing instead of watching TV.

Motivating tips

- Choose exercises and activities that you enjoy.

- Pick a convenient time and place for your exercise.

- Don't worry if you weigh more for the first few months. You are most likely replacing fat tissue with muscle. Muscle weighs more than fat.

- Check your measurements with a tape measure. You'll be able to see that you're getting leaner.

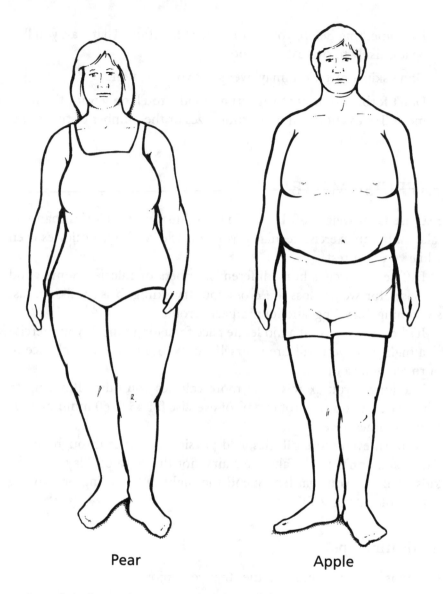

Pear   Apple

People who carry more weight on the hips and thighs are pear-shaped. People who carry more weight around the waist and abdomen are apple-shaped. Apple-shaped people are more likely to have blood vessel disease, heart disease, high blood pressure, high blood fat levels, insulin resistance, and poor blood glucose control.

HOW TO KEEP THE WEIGHT OFF

When you have reached your ideal body weight, the hard part comes. Keeping weight off is much more difficult than losing it.

Most people will regain lost weight. Many people gain back even more weight than they lost. This happens because people return to their old eating and exercise habits after they lose weight.

To maintain your ideal body weight, keep up your new habits. Don't go back to your old ones. If you do, you'll gain back all the weight you worked so hard to lose.

Index

Other Books by the American Diabetes Association

Self-Care Titles

NEW!

Dear Diabetes Advisor

This book offers plain and simple answers to several questions about diabetes. Written in an easy-to-understand format, you'll discover all you need to know about treatment, exercise, healthy cooking and eating, weight loss, insurance, and more.

Softcover. #CSMDDA
Nonmember: $9.95/ADA Member: $8.95

NEW!

Type 2 Diabetes: Your Healthy Living Guide, Second Edition

A thorough guide to staying healthy with type 2 diabetes—everything from choosing a health care team and eating and exercising to self-monitoring, insulin, dealing with complications, and keeping mentally fit. You'll also find tips on employment and health insurance.

Softcover. #CTIIHG
Nonmember: $16.95/ADA Member: $14.95

NEW!

The Ten Keys to Helping Your Child Grow Up With Diabetes

Here's help for parents who face the problems, feelings, and situations that can accompany managing diabetes. *Ten Keys* is a practical book for parents and caregivers of children with diabetes that addresses in detail the psychological, social, and emotional hurdles that often complicate the lives of youngsters with diabetes.

Softcover. #CSMTK
Nonmember: $14.95/ADA Member: $13.95

NEW!

Women & Diabetes

Designed for women, and filled with complete, thorough, and up-to-date discussions about a broad range of real-life topics such PMS, lactation, sex, pregnancy, child rearing, and menopause. Also includes dozens of checklists, charts, and exercises to help you create an individualized roadmap to living a healthy life with diabetes.

Softcover. #CSMWD
Nonmember: $14.95/ADA Member: $13.95

NEW!

Caring for the Diabetic Soul

You'll learn about coping with denial, controlling your stress and anger, building self-esteem, and much more. Written by professionals whose lives have been touched by diabetes—nurses, counselors, professors, doctors, and parents—each chapter reflects a personal experience that will touch you, too. Softcover. #CSMCDS

Nonmember: $9.95/ADA Member: $8.95

American Diabetes Association Complete Guide to Diabetes

Every area of self-care is covered in this ultimate diabetes reference for your home. With it, you can solve problems with hundreds of hints, tips, and tricks that are proven to work. It covers insulin use. Blood sugar control. Sex and pregnancy. Eating and weight control. Insurance. Mastering diabetes supplies. Every aspect of your daily and professional life. You'll turn to this all-in-one guide again and again!

Hardcover. #CSMCGD
Nonmember: $29.95/ADA Member: $25.95

NEW!
Softcover. #CSMCGDP
Nonmember: $19.95/ADA Member: $17.95

101 Tips for Staying Healthy with Diabetes

Get the inside track on the latest tips, techniques, and strategies for preventing and treating diabetes complications. You'll learn how to treat and prevent skin infections, which cold and flu medicines to avoid, and how to eat the foods you like healthfully.

Softcover. #CSMFSH
Nonmember: $12.95/ADA Member: $10.95

How to Get Great Diabetes Care

This book explains the ADA Standards of Care and informs you of the importance of seeking medical attention that meets these standards. Includes discussions on the different types of diabetes, the goals of treatment, how to choose and effectively talk to your doctor, and more.

Softcover. #CSMHGGDC
Nonmember: $11.95/ADA Member: $9.95

Sweet Kids: How to Balance Diabetes Control & Good Nutrition with Family Peace

This new guide addresses behavioral and developmental issues of nutrition management in the families of children with diabetes. Each chapter begins with a story of a child with diabetes to help introduce you to each of the book's topics.

Softcover. #CSMSK
Nonmember: $14.95/ADA Member: $11.95

Reflections on Diabetes

A collection of stories written by people who have learned from the experience of living with the disease. Selected from the *Reflections* column of *Diabetes Forecast* magazine.

Softcover. #CSMROD
Nonmember: $9.95/ADA Member: $8.95

101 Tips for Improving Your Blood Sugar

101 Tips offers a practical, easy-to-follow roadmap to tight blood sugar control. One question appears on each page, with the answers or "tips" below each question. Tips on diet, exercise, travel, weight loss, insulin, illness, and more.

Softcover. #CSMTBBGC
Nonmember: $12.95/ADA Member: $10.95

Managing Diabetes on a Budget

For less than $10 you can begin saving hundreds and hundreds on your diabetes self-care. An inexpensive, sure-fire collection of tips and hints to save you money on everything from medications and diet to exercise and health care.

Softcover. #CSMMDOAB
Nonmember: $7.95/ADA Member: $6.95

The Fitness Book: For People with Diabetes

You'll learn how to exercise to lose weight, exercise safely, increase your competitive edge, get your mind and body ready to exercise, much more.

Softcover. #CSMFB
Nonmember: $18.95/ADA Member: $16.95

Raising a Child with Diabetes

Learn how to help your child adjust insulin to allow for foods kids like to eat, have a busy schedule and still feel healthy and strong, negotiate the twists and turns of being "different," and much more.

Softcover. #CSMRACWD
Nonmember: $14.95/ADA Member: $12.95

The Dinosaur Tamer

Enjoy 25 fictional stories that will entertain, enlighten, and ease your child's frustrations about having diabetes. Each tale warmly evaporates the fear of insulin shots, blood tests, going to diabetes camp, and more. Ages 8–12.

Softcover. #CSMDTAOS
Nonmember: $9.95/ADA Member: $8.95

Grilled Cheese at Four O'Clock in the Morning

Your child's fears and frustrations of having diabetes will be eased when they read about Scott, a young boy who develops diabetes.

Softcover. #CCHGC
Nonmember: $6.95/ ADA Member: $5.95

The Take-Charge Guide to Type I Diabetes

Discover how to prevent complications, increase your chances of having a healthy baby, learn all you can from testing your blood sugar, much more.

Softcover. #CSMT1
Nonmember: $16.95/ADA Member: $13.50

Diabetes & Pregnancy: What to Expect

You'll learn about an unborn baby's development, tests to expect, labor and delivery, birth control, much more.

Softcover. #CPREDP
Nonmember: $9.95/ADA Member: $8.95

Gestational Diabetes: What to Expect

Discover what gestational diabetes is and how to care for yourself during your pregnancy. You'll learn about an unborn baby's development, tests to expect, labor and delivery, birth control, much more.

Softcover. #CPREGD
Nonmember: $9.95/ADA Member: $8.95

Necessary Toughness

You'll be inspired by this story of an athlete with the courage to face not only NFL linemen but also the threat of diabetes. You'll learn that you *can* live a healthy, happy life.

Softcover. #CGFNT
Nonmember: $7.95/ADA Member: $6.95

Diabetes: A Positive Approach—Video

#CVIDPOS
Nonmember: $19.95/ADA Member: $17.95

Cookbooks & Meal Planners

NEW!
The Diabetes Carbohydrate and Fat Gram Guide

Calories are important, but knowing the fat and carbohydrate content of the foods you eat is the key to eating right. Registered dietitian Lea Ann Holzmeister shows you how to count carbohydrate and fat grams and exchanges, and why it's important. Dozens of charts list foods, serving sizes, and nutrient data for hundreds of products.

Softcover. #CMPCFGG
Nonmember: $11.95/ADA Member: $9.95

NEW!
Brand-Name Diabetic Meals in Minutes

Save time cooking with these popular taste-tested recipes from the kitchens of Campbell Soup, Kraft Foods, Weetabix, Dean Foods, Eskimo Pie, and Equal. Features more than 200 recipes from appetizers to desserts that will help make your meals tastier and your life easier. Nutrient information included. Softcover. #CCBBNDM
Nonmember: $12.95/ADA Member: $10.95

NEW!
How to Cook for People with Diabetes

Finally, a collection of reader favorites from the delicious, nutritious recipes featured every month in *Diabetes Forecast*. But you don't only get ideas for pizza, chicken, unique holiday foods, vegetarian recipes and more, you also get nutrient analysis and exchanges for each recipe.

Softcover. #CCBCFPD
Nonmember: $11.95/ADA Member: $9.95

NEW!

Magic Menus

Now you can plan all your meals from more than 50 breakfasts, 50 lunches, 75 dinners, and 30 snacks. Like magic, this book figures fats, calories, and exchanges for you automatically. The day's calories will still equal 1,500. Thousands of combinations are possible.

Softcover. #CCBMM
Nonmember: $14.95/ADA Member: $12.95

NEW!

World-Class Diabetic Cooking

Travel around the world at every meal with a collection of 200 exciting new low-fat, low-calorie recipes. Features recipes from Thailand, Italy, Greece, Spain, China, Japan, Africa, Mexico, Germany, and more. Appetizers, soups, salads, pastas, meats, breads, and desserts are highlighted.

Softcover. #CCBWCC
Nonmember: $12.95/ADA Member: $10.95

NEW!

Southern-Style Diabetic Cooking

This cookbook takes traditional Southern dishes and turns them into great-tasting recipes you'll come back to again and again. Features more than 100 recipes including appetizers, main dishes, and desserts; complete nutrient analysis with each recipe, and suggestions for modifying recipes to meet individual nutritional needs.

Softcover. #CCBSSDC
Nonmember: $11.95/ADA Member: $9.95

Flavorful Seasons Cookbook

Warm up your winter with recipes for Christmas, welcome spring with an Easter recipe, and cool off those hot summer days with more recipes for the Fourth of July. More than 400 unforgettable choices that combine great taste with all the good-for-you benefits of a well-balanced meal. Cornish Game Hens, Orange Sea Bass, Ginger Bread Pudding, many others.

Softcover. #CCBFS
Nonmember: $16.95/ADA Member: $14.95

Diabetic Meals In 30 Minutes—Or Less!

Put an end to bland, time-consuming meals with more than 140 fast, flavorful recipes. Complete nutrition information accompanies every recipe. A number of "quick tips" will have you out of the kitchen and into the dining room even faster! Salsa Salad, Oven-Baked Parmesan Zucchini, Roasted Red Pepper Soup, Layered Vanilla Parfait, and more.

Softcover. #CCBDM
Nonmember: $11.95/ADA Member: $9.95

Diabetes Meal Planning Made Easy

Learn quick and easy ways to eat more starches, fruits, vegetables, and milk; make changes in your eating habits to reach your goals; and understand how to use the Nutrition Facts on food labels. You'll also master the intricacies of each food group in the new Diabetes Food Pyramid.

Softcover. #CCBMP
Nonmember: $14.95/ADA Member: $12.95

Month of Meals

When celebrations begin, go ahead—dig in! Includes a Special Occasion section that offers tips for brunches, holidays, and restaurants to give you a delicious dining options anytime, anywhere. Menu choices include Chicken Cacciatore, Oven Fried Fish, Sloppy Joes, Crab Cakes, and many others.

Softcover. #CMPMOM
Nonmember: $12.50/ADA Member: $10.50

Month of Meals 2

Automatic menu planning goes ethnic! Tips and meal suggestions for Mexican, Italian, and Chinese restaurants are featured. Quick-to-fix and ethnic recipes are also included. Beef Burritos, Chop Suey, Veal Piccata, Stuffed Peppers, and others.

Softcover. #CMPMOM2
Nonmember: $12.50/ADA Member: $10.50

Month of Meals 3

Enjoy fast food without guilt! Make delicious choices at McDonald's, Wendy's, Taco Bell, and other fast food restaurants. Special sections offer valuable tips such as reading ingredient labels, preparing meals for picnics, and meal planning when you're ill.

Softcover. #CMPMOM3
Nonmember: $12.50/ADA Member: $10.50

Month of Meals 4

Meat and potatoes menu planning! Enjoy with old-time family favorites like Meatloaf and Pot Roast, Crispy Fried Chicken, Beef Stroganoff, and many others. Hints for turning family-size meals into delicious left-overs will keep generous portions from going to waste. Meal plans for one or two people are also featured. Spiral-bound.

Softcover. #CMPMOM4
Nonmember: $12.50/ADA Member: $10.50

Month of Meals 5

Meatless meals picked fresh from the garden. Choose from a garden of fresh vegetarian selections like Eggplant Italian, Stuffed Zucchini, Cucumbers with Dill Dressing, Vegetable Lasagna, and many others. Plus, you'll reap all the health benefits of a vegetarian diet.

Softcover. #CMPMOM5
Nonmember: $12.50/ADA Member: $10.50

Great Starts & Fine Finishes

Try Crab-Filled Mushrooms, Broiled Shrimp or Baked Scallops for an appetizer. Dig into Cherry Cobbler or Chocolate Chip Cookies for dessert.

Softcover. #CCBGSFF
Nonmember: $8.95/ADA Member: $7.15

Easy & Elegant Entrees

Enjoy Fettucini with Peppers and Broccoli, Steak and Brandied Onions, Shrimp Creole, many more. You'll also enjoy peace of mind knowing your meals are low in fat and calories.

Softcover. #CCBEEE
Nonmember: $8.95/ADA Member: $7.15

Savory Soups & Salads

Pasta-Stuffed Tomato Salad, Mediterranean Chicken Salad, Seafood Salad, many others. Hungry for soup? Try a bowl of Clam Chowder, Gazpacho, Mushroom and Barley, others.

Softcover. #CCBSSS
Nonmember: $8.95/ADA Member: $7.15

Quick & Hearty Main Dishes

Try Spicy Chicken Drumsticks, Apple Cinnamon Pork Chops, Chicken and Turkey Burgers, Macaroni and Cheese, Beef Stroganoff, and dozens more.

Softcover. #CCBQHMD
Nonmember: $8.95/ADA Member: $7.15

Simple & Tasty Side Dishes

Sauted Sweet Peppers, Onion-Seasoned Rice, Parsley-Stuffed Potatoes, Brown Rice with Mushrooms, Broccoli with Lemon Butter Sauce, and a pantry of others.

Softcover. #CCBSTSD
Nonmember: $8.95/ADA Member: $7.15

How to Order

1. **To order by phone:** just call us at **1-800-232-6733** and have your credit card ready. VISA, MasterCard, and American Express are accepted. Please mention code **CK997AZ** when ordering.

2. **To order by mail:** on a separate sheet of paper, write down the books you're ordering and calculate the total using the shipping & handling chart below. (NOTE: Virginia residents add 4.5% sales tax; Georgia residents add 6.0% sales tax.) Then include your check, written to the American Diabetes Association, with your order and mail to:

American Diabetes Association
Order Fulfillment Department
P.O. Box 930850
Atlanta, GA 31193-0850

Shipping & Handling Chart

up to $30.00. . . . . add $4.00

$30.01–$50.00 . . . . . . add $5.00

over $50.00 . . . . add 10%

Allow 2–3 weeks for shipment. Add $4.00 to shipping & handling for each extra shipping address. Add $15 for each overseas shipment. Prices subject to change without notice.

About the
American Diabetes Association

The American Diabetes Association is the nation's leading voluntary health organization supporting diabetes research, information, and advocacy. Founded in 1940, the Association provides services to communities across the country. Its mission is to prevent and cure diabetes and to improve the lives of all people affected by diabetes.

For more than 50 years, the American Diabetes Association has been the leading publisher of comprehensive diabetes information for people with diabetes and the health care professionals who treat them. Its huge library of practical and authoritative books for people with diabetes covers every aspect of self-care—cooking and nutrition, fitness, weight control, medications, complications, emotional issues, and general self care. The Association also publishes books and medical treatment guides for physicians and other health care professionals.

Membership in the Association is available to health care professionals and people with diabetes and includes subscriptions to one or more of the Association's periodicals. People with diabetes receive *Diabetes Forecast*, the nation's leading health and wellness magazine for people with diabetes. Health care professionals receive one or more of the Association's five scientific and medical journals.

For more information, please call toll-free:

Questions about diabetes:	1-800-DIABETES
Membership, people with diabetes:	1-800-806-7801
Membership, health professionals:	1-800-232-3472
Free catalog of ADA books:	1-800-232-6733
Visit us on the Web:	www.diabetes.org